BOY SCOUTS OF AMERICA®

Be Prepared
First
Aid

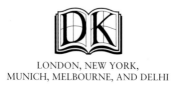

LONDON, NEW YORK,
MUNICH, MELBOURNE, AND DELHI

Boy Scouts of America ® and Be Prepared ® are registered
trademarks of the Boy Scouts of America. Printed under
license from Boy Scouts of America to DK Publishing.
www.scouting.org

The material in this book reflects current first-aid practice at the time of publication but
cannot be a substitute for actual training.

For convenience and clarity, we have used the pronoun "he" when referring to the first
aider or victim, unless the individual in the accompanying photograph is female.

This edition published in the United States in 2007 by

DK Publishing
375 Hudson Street
New York, New York 10014

A Penguin Company

07 08 09 10 11   10 9 8 7 6 5 4 3 2 1
Copyright © 2007 Dorling Kindersley Limited, London
Text copyright © 2007 The British Red Cross Society

A CIP catalogue record for this book is available from the Library of Congress

ISBN: 978-0-7566-3521-3

DK books are available at special discounts when purchased in bulk for sales promotions,
premiums, fund-raising, or educational use. For details, contact DK Publishing Special
Markets, 375 Hudson Street, New York, New York 10014 or SpecialSales@dk.com

Color reproduction by GRB Editrice, Italy
Printed and bound by L. Rex Printing Co Ltd, China

Discover more at
www.dk.com

Contents

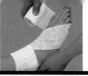

Boy Scouts of America

The mission of the Boys Scouts of America is to prepare young people to make ethical and moral choices over their lifetimes by instilling in them the values of the Scout Oath and Law. The programs of the Boy Scouts of America—Cub Scouting, Boy Scouting, Varsity Scouting, and Venturing—pursue these aims through methods designed for the age and maturity of the participants.

Cub Scouting: A family- and home-centered program for boys in the first through fifth grade (or 7, 8, 9, and 10 years old). Cub Scouting's emphasis is on quality programs at the local level, where the most boys and families are involved. Fourth- and fifth-grade (or 10-year-old) boys are called Webelos (WE'll BE LOyal Scouts) and participate in more advanced activities that begin to prepare them to become Boy Scouts.

Boy Scouting: A program for boys 11 through 17 designed to acheive the aims of Scouting through a vigorous outdoor program and peer group leadership with the counsel of an adult Scoutmaster. (Boys may also become Boy Scouts if they have earned the Arrow of Light Award or have completed the fifth grade.)

Varsity Scouting: An active, exciting program for young men 14 through 17 built around five program fields of emphasis: advancement, high adventure, personal development, service, and special programs, and events.

Venturing: This is for young men and young women ages 14 through 20. It includes challenging high-adventure activities, sports, and hobbies for teenagers that teach leadership skills, provide opportunities to teach others, and to learn and grow in a supporting, caring, and fun environment.

For more on Scouting programs visit www.scouting.org

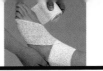

Introduction

First Aid is the initial help that is given to someone who is injured or suddenly taken ill. Knowing how to treat a victim in the first moments after an event can make all the difference. Some of the techniques in this book will help make a victim comfortable until assistance arrives, other techniques can potentially save lives. First Aid is as relevant at home as on high-adventure activities. This book provides advice for a variety of injuries and conditions, some of which can be safely delivered by any level of Scout, others are aimed at the older age groups; the suitable levels are indicated at the bottom of each page of the book.

Easy-to-follow guide

Be Prepared: First Aid provides instant access to essential first-aid techniques for every emergency from how to give life-saving first aid to an unconscious person, to treating a blister, or removing a splinter. The book is divided into eight color-coded chapters, according to the type of injury and, for easy access to the informaton, every technique is set in a separate color panel.

Essential information

There is useful backgound information on how you should approach an incident to ensure both your own safety as well as that of the victim. You are shown how to assess a victim and carry out a head-to-toe survey and there is advice on how to call the most appropriate assistance from the emergency services. The book also details what to keep in a first aid kit, whether for the home or for an expedition, as well as providing essential step-by-step guidelines for applying the dressings and bandages.

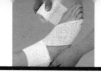

How to use this book

Be prepared: first aid clearly links theory to practice. It has eight sections, arranged by type of injury or condition. Throughout there are realistic "incidents" photographed in the home, outdoors, or in the workplace that show you what to do in an emergency. In addition, every section ends with a "Test yourself" panel to reinforce new learning. This book may be used as a companion guide to support rank advancement within the Cub Scouting, Boy Scouting, Venturing, or Sea Scouting programs of the Boy Scouts of America. Please check the most current program handbook for specific requirements.

Emergency first-aid incidents
Each section of the book has a realistic incident showing how to put the guidance into practice

"What you should do" box outlines the first-aid action you should take in clearly identified steps

"Important" box highlights principal do's and don't's to enable you to give successful first aid

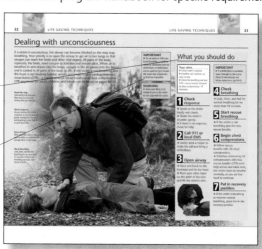

First-aid treatments
Every illness or injury is presented in a separate color panel so that you can find information quickly and easily

"Your aims" and "You will need" boxes outline your treatment priorities and essential equipment

Step-by-step headings tell you exactly what you should do

"Signs and symptoms" help you confirm the victim's injury

"Warning" box advises urgent action you may need to take

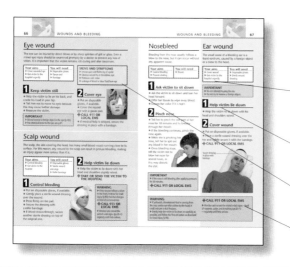

1 First-aid principles

This chapter explains the essentials that every first aider needs to know when dealing with an emergency. It sets out how you should deal with every aspect of an incident, from the importance of ensuring your own and other people's safety, to finding the most appropriate bandage or sling to put on an injury.

There are clear guidelines for dealing with any type of emergency, from rescuing a drowning victim to managing a major incident with multiple casualties. Easy-to-follow charts and step-by-step instructions throughout show you how to assess a victim's condition, summon help, and monitor a victim while waiting for help to arrive.

Use the questionnaire on page 30 to test your understanding of your role as a first aider and your knowledge of first-aid materials.

Contents

Dealing with an incident

Faced with an incident, first make sure that the area is safe, then assess any injuries; after that, decide what action to take. Whatever the situation, stay calm and confident to reassure the victims. If you are sure that the scene of the incident is safe, try to locate all the victims; some may have been thrown some distance or wandered away. If there is

> **WARNING**
> ▶ If sure you are not putting yourself in danger when approaching an incident. If vehicles are involved, look in particular for smoke, fire, and hazardous chemicals (p.10).
> ▶ If there is an unconscious victim, be ready to begin resuscitation if necessary (pp.36–52).

more than one victim, decide who is the most seriously injured (see Dealing with more than one victim p.14) and treat him first. Ask bystanders to help with the less seriously injured.

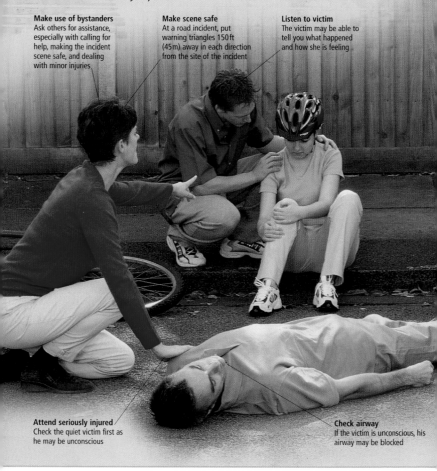

Make use of bystanders
Ask others for assistance, especially with calling for help, making the incident scene safe, and dealing with minor injuries

Make scene safe
At a road incident, put warning triangles 150 ft (45 m) away in each direction from the site of the incident

Listen to victim
The victim may be able to tell you what happened and how she is feeling

Attend seriously injured
Check the quiet victim first as he may be unconscious

Check airway
If the victim is unconscious, his airway may be blocked

Get help
Call the emergency services. Ideally, ask a bystander to do this

What you should do

Your aims
▶ Deal with any danger
▶ Assess incident
▶ Call emergency services
▶ Get help from others
▶ Give emergency first aid

IMPORTANT
▶ If there are obvious dangers, wait for the emergency services to arrive—do not approach the scene until they tell you it is safe. Keep bystanders away.

1 Make area safe

● Check for danger as you approach the incident.
● If it is safe to do so, assess any victims.
● If it is not safe, or if it is a major incident, such as a multiple car accident or a fire, call 911 or local EMS.

2 Assess victims

● Determine how many victims are involved.
● Assess who is most seriously injured—attend to quiet victims first, as they may be unconscious.
● Carry out an initial assessment of the victims (p.16).
● If any victim is unconscious, be ready to begin resuscitation (pp.36–52).

3 Get help

● If any victim is seriously injured, call 911 or your local EMS—tell the dispatcher how many victims there are.
● If possible, ask a bystander to make the call.

4 Give emergency aid

● If a victim is conscious, carry out a detailed assessment (p.17).
● Treat life-threatening injuries such as severe bleeding before minor injuries such as sprains.
● Ask bystanders to help the less seriously injured or gather equipment.

5 Monitor casualties

● Monitor and record the victims' vital signs—level of response, pulse, and breathing (pp.20–1)—regularly until help arrives.
● Pass the information you record on to the emergency services.

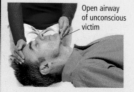
Open airway of unconscious victim

Treat victims where found
Leave the victims where they are and give them emergency aid. Do not move them unless there is further danger

Assessing dangers

In an emergency, you must make sure that by approaching an incident or a victim, you are not putting your own life at risk. Stay calm, use common sense, take precautions to avoid the risk of cross infection, and follow a plan to help you deal with casualties effectively.

Dealing with a road incident

At any road incident, you need to make the area safe before giving first aid. Make sure you are not putting yourself at risk by approaching the victim when there is any danger. You need to protect yourself, any victims, and other road users. Use a flashlight.

1 Call emergency services

- Park your vehicle, switch on flashing hazard lights, and call 911 or local EMS.

2 Warn others

- Set up warning triangles. Place them in the road at least 150ft (45m) away from the site of the incident in each direction.
- Send helpers to warn other drivers.
- Never cross a busy highway.

3 Identify hazards

- Look for any hazards, such as vehicles with hazardous substance panels.
- Stabilize any vehicles; turn off the ignition and put on the handbrake.

4 Check for casualties

- Check for casualties who may have been thrown some distance from a car or wandered away in shock.

Rescuing a victim from water

Incidents around water often involve people who have fallen into, or have been swimming in, cold water or strong currents. Do not endanger your life when attempting rescue.

1 Call emergency services

- If possible, ask a bystander to call 911.

2 Rescue from water's edge

- Lie down at the water's edge so that you do not get pulled into the water.
- Throw a rope or float to the victim, or reach out with a stick or branch.

3 If you have to go into water

- To make sure that you remain safe, wade rather than swim, and do not go out of your depth.
- Lift the victim out of the water.

4 Keep victim warm

- Try to shield the victim from wind to help prevent him from becoming colder.
- Treat for hypothermia if necessary (p.86).
- Take or send the victim to the hospital, even if he appears to have recovered.

IMPORTANT
☐ If the victim is unconscious, lift him out of the water with his head lower than his chest, to prevent fluid from entering his airway if he vomits.

Electrical injuries

Injuries caused by electricity most commonly occur in the home as a result of contact with a low-voltage domestic current, usually due to faulty switches or appliances. Contact with electricity can cause serious injury or even death because the current passes through the body, causing burns and sometimes stopping the heart from beating. Contact with high-voltage electricity (below) is usually fatal.

1 Switch off current

● Break the electrical contact by switching off the current.

IMPORTANT
☐ Do not touch the victim if he is still in contact with the electricity, he may be "live".

2 Separate victim from electrical source

● If you cannot switch off the current, stand on some dry insulating material, such as a plastic mat, a folded newspaper, or a book such as a telephone directory.
● If you know it is safe you can use something wooden to push the victim away from the source of the electricity or push the source from him. Do not use anything metallic.
● If you cannot separate the victim from the electrical source, loop rope around his ankles and pull him away from the source.

Push electrical source away with dry wood such as a wooden broom handle

WARNING
☐ If the victim is unconscious,

✚ CALL 911 OR LOCAL EMS

Open the airway and check breathing (p.37). Put him in the recovery position if he is breathing. Be ready to begin CPR if necessary (pp.36–52).

3 Treat burns

● If the victim is conscious, check for burns and treat accordingly (p.82).

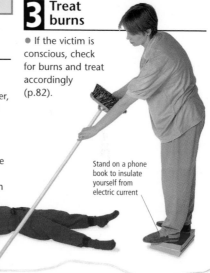

Stand on a phone book to insulate yourself from electric current

High-voltage electricity

This is the type found in overhead power lines and high-tension cables. Anyone who survives contact will suffer serious burns.
● Call the emergency services.
● Ask for help from electrical engineers to shut off the power.
● Do not approach or allow anyone else to approach the victim until you are certain that the power has been cut off and isolated. Everyone should stay at least 60ft (18m) away, as high-voltage electricity can jump ("arc") this distance.
● When you are officially told it is safe to do so, assess the victim.
● Be ready to begin resuscitation if necessary (pp.36–52).

Dealing with a fire

If a smoke alarm gives you warning of smoke or a fire, evacuate the building quickly. When fire breaks out, it is essential to think quickly and clearly because flames and smoke can spread rapidly. Alert the emergency services and warn anyone who may be in danger.

WARNING
▶ Do not use the elevator in any circumstances.
▶ Do not open a door without first touching the door or handle with the back of your hand to see if it is hot. Heat indicates fire behind the door, so choose a different escape route.

1 Raise alarm

● In a public building, activate the nearest fire alarm and warn other people who are at risk.
● Call 911.

2 Assess danger

● If the fire has taken hold, do not attempt to put it out yourself.
● If the fire is small, you discover it early, and you have a fire blanket or fire extinguisher, try to smother the flames. If you cannot extinguish the fire within 30 seconds, leave the building.

IMPORTANT
▶ If trapped by fire, go into a room with a window and shut the door. Open the window and call for help. If escaping through a window, go out feet first. Lower yourself by your arms before dropping to the ground.

3 Get to safety

● If you are in a large building, follow the marked escape routes and help others, especially those who are vulnerable, such as children and elderly people.
● Close all doors behind you.
● Walk quickly and calmly—do not run.
● Do not enter a smoke-filled room.
● If you do need to cross a smoky area, try to stay close to the ground where the air will be clearer.

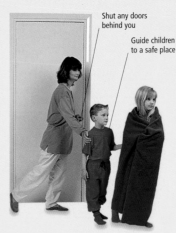

Shut any doors behind you

Guide children to a safe place

If a victim's clothing is on fire

● Stop the victim from running around.
● Drop him to the ground.
● Wrap him in heavy fabric, such as a wool or cotton blanket.
● Roll the victim gently along the ground until the flames are extinguished.
● Do not use anything synthetic to try to put out the fire.

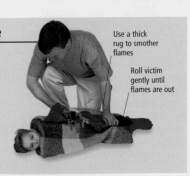

Use a thick rug to smother flames

Roll victim gently until flames are out

Avoiding cross infection

It is possible to be infected with certain viruses, such as HIV (human immunodeficiency virus) and hepatitis B or C, through contact with the blood or other body fluids of an infected person. Handle a victim's body fluids as hygienically as possible to keep the risk of any cross infection to a minimum. Avoid germs being transmitted when giving rescue breaths by using a special face mask (p.23). This is a plastic barrier with a filter that helps protect against contact with body fluids.

> **IMPORTANT**
> ▶ If gloves are unavailable, you must still give life-saving treatment.
> ▶ If your eyes, nose, mouth, or any wound on your skin is splashed by the victim's blood, wash thoroughly with water immediately and consult a doctor as soon as possible.

Wash hands

Whenever possible, wash your hands thoroughly before and after treating a victim. Make sure you wash the back and front of your hands.

Wear gloves

Whenever possible, put on disposable gloves. If you do not have any gloves, you can protect your hands with clean plastic bags.

Cover wound

When you cover a wound with a dressing, do not touch the inside sterile pad of the dressing. If possible, wear disposable gloves when applying dressings.

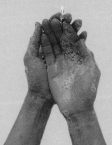
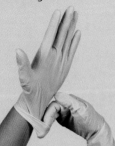
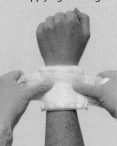

Removing waste

Once you have finished treatment, dispose of all waste carefully to prevent the spread of infection. Use plastic bags or, if you have them, special red biohazard bags. For sharp objects, use specially designed red boxes called sharp object containers.

● Sharp object containers are used for the disposal of needles and any other sharp objects. They must be collected and disposed of by authorized collectors.

Sharp object container

● Biohazard bags are designed for the disposal of soiled dressings and other waste products. They should be securely sealed and incinerated.

Keep gloves on while disposing of waste and then put them in bag

Disposal bag

Managing an incident

At the scene of an incident, adopt a systematic approach, since there is likely to be confusion. Make sure the area is safe and contact the emergency services. You should be clear about dealing with multiple victims and always enlist help from bystanders.

Dealing with more than one victim

In situations such as car accidents, you may find yourself dealing with several victims. Whether you are working alone or with others, it is vital to stay calm.

1 Assess victims

- Make sure area is safe. Perform primary surveys (p.16) to identify victims who have life-threatening injuries.
- Check quiet victims first as they may be unconscious.
- Enlist help to move victims with minor injuries quickly from the site and allow access to serious cases.

2 Attend to unconscious victims

- Prioritize the treatment of any unconscious victims.

3 Treat conscious victims

- Treat conscious victims with serious injuries first.
- Treat victims with minor injuries.

Moving a victim

- Do not move a victim to give first aid unless it is safe for you to approach, he is in immediate danger, and you have the correct training and equipment.

- You may need to move a victim if: he is in danger of drowning; he is at risk due to fire, smoke, a bomb, or gunfire; or he is in or near a collapsing building.

Getting help from others

You may be faced with several tasks at the scene of the incident, such as maintaining safety, calling for help, and starting first aid. Bystanders may be able to assist you.

1 Give clear instructions

- Let everyone know at the scene of an incident that you are trained in first aid.
- Be clear with bystanders about what you want them to do.
- You may want to ask bystanders to: locate victims; call the emergency services; control traffic and onlookers; bring first-aid equipment; maintain a victim's privacy; or help with first aid.

2 Follow through

- If you do send a bystander to call for help, see that he returns to confirm that the call has been made.
- If other first aiders come forward, give them as much information as possible. The most senior first aider present should take charge of the team.
- When the emergency services arrive, they will take control.

Getting appropriate help

Help in an emergency is available from a variety of services. In most areas, dialling 911 free from any phone (including cell phones) will put you through to a dispatcher who will connect you to the police or fire department or EMS (emergency medical service). If your area has a different number you should keep a note of it. Some large organizations also have their own arrangments for call the emergency services.

Throughout this book, advice is given on the type of medical help to seek. There are three main categories as follows:

✚ **GET MEDICAL HELP**
when advice about treatment is necessary.

✚ **TAKE OR SEND VICTIM TO THE HOSPITAL**
when hospital treatment is essential. You may be able to take the victim yourself.

✚ **CALL 911 OR LOCAL EMS**
when urgent treatment is needed.

Calling the emergency services

When you dial 911, you will be asked which service you need. If there are victims ask for the EMS. Speak calmly and clearly. Give the following details:
● Your phone number.
● The location of the incident.
● The type and seriousness of the incident, for example, "One car overturned, two victims trapped".

● The number of victims and details of injury— "One male with breathing difficulties."
● Details of hazards such as chemicals.
● Do not hang up until told to.

Coping with stress

An emergency can be very distressing for everyone involved. To safeguard your own welfare and remain effective as a first aider, recognize that feelings of stress are normal.

1 Be prepared for reaction

● Realize that it is natural to feel stressed about giving first aid and to be emotional after you have finished treating a victim.
● You might feel satisfied at having done a good job, confused about whether you did the "right things," or angry and sad if the outcome of the incident is upsetting.

2 Watch for symptoms

● Stress may manifest itself in any of the following symptoms: tremor of the hands and stomach; excessive sweating; flashbacks; nightmares or disturbed sleep; tearfulness; tension and irritability; or a feeling of withdrawal and isolation.

3 Talk about feelings

● To help you face up to your emotions, talk about how you feel with a friend and/ or your parents. By releasing your feelings as soon after the event as possible, you should find yourself able to cope more easily.

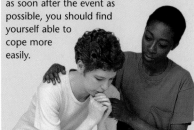

IMPORTANT
▶ If you are experiencing symptoms of stress and they do not pass in time, or if you are concerned, seek further advice from your doctor.

Initial assessment of a victim

Your priority when attending a victim is to assess him for life-threatening conditions, such as lack of breathing, that need urgent first aid. Carry out a more detailed assessment (opposite) only when you have established that the victim is breathing normally.

Primary survey

This initial assessment involves looking for danger to yourself and the victim, checking whether the victim is conscious and breathing (and beginning cardiopulmonary resuscitation—CPR—if necessary). Detailed guidelines for life-saving sequences for adults, children, and infants can be found on pages 36–52.

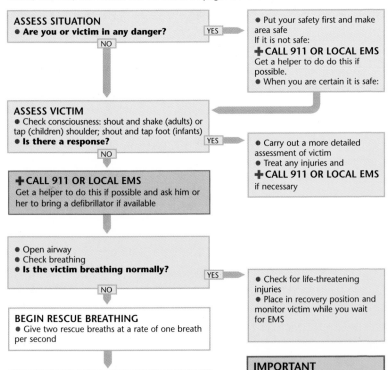

ASSESS SITUATION
● **Are you or victim in any danger?** | YES |
| NO |

● Put your safety first and make area safe
If it is not safe:
✚ **CALL 911 OR LOCAL EMS**
Get a helper to do do this if possible.
● When you are certain it is safe:

ASSESS VICTIM
● Check consciousness: shout and shake (adults) or tap (children) shoulder; shout and tap foot (infants)
● **Is there a response?** | YES |
| NO |

● Carry out a more detailed assessment of victim
● Treat any injuries and
✚ **CALL 911 OR LOCAL EMS**
if necessary

✚ **CALL 911 OR LOCAL EMS**
Get a helper to do this if possible and ask him or her to bring a defibrillator if available

● Open airway
● Check breathing
● **Is the victim breathing normally?** | YES |
| NO |

● Check for life-threatening injuries
● Place in recovery position and monitor victim while you wait for EMS

BEGIN RESCUE BREATHING
● Give two rescue breaths at a rate of one breath per second

BEGIN CHEST COMPRESSIONS
● Give 30 chest compressions at a rate of 100 per minute
● Repeat two more rescue breaths
● Continue alternating chest compressions and rescue breaths 30:2 (cardiopulmonary resuscitation/CPR) until emergency help arrives, the victim starts to breathe normally, or you are too exhausted to keep going

IMPORTANT
▶ If you are on your own and the the victim is a child, give CPR for two minutes (about five cycles) before you call 911 or local EMS.

Detailed assessment of a victim

Once the victim is out of danger, you have completed the primary survey, and no further life-saving actions are needed, carry out a detailed assessment of the victim, known as a secondary survey, to find out more about the victim's condition. If a victim complains of a particular problem, treat this first. You also need to monitor the victim's vital signs—level of response, pulse, and breathing (pp.20–21).

> **Your aims**
> ▶ Obtain full history of incident by questioning victim or onlookers
> ▶ Find out more about circumstances in which injury was sustained and forces involved—this is known as the mechanics of injury
> ▶ Assess general signs and symptoms—find out how victim is feeling and how serious his condition is
> ▶ Examine victim thoroughly—look for details of victim's condition that you can see, feel, hear, or smell

Taking a history of the incident

Try to form a full picture of the situation by asking the following questions:

● What happened?
How did the problem occur? Has the victim had this problem before? Does anything make it better or worse?
● When did it happen?
What time did the problem start? Was the victim doing anything in particular?
● Where did it happen?
Was the victim in a particular environment when the problem started? Were there any hazards in the area?

● Why did it happen?
Does the victim know why it happened? Were there any factors in the area that might have contributed to the problem?

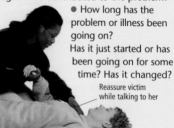

● How long has the problem or illness been going on?
Has it just started or has been going on for some time? Has it changed?

Reassure victim while talking to her

Finding out how the incident happened

You may be able to gain more clues about potential injuries by looking to see how an incident has happened. For example:
● If a victim falls from a height of over 6ft (2m), he is likely to sustain severe injuries, such as pelvic fractures, spinal injuries, and damage to internal organs.
● In a vehicle incident, a victim who is hit from the side is likely to sustain more severe injuries than if he is hit from the front. This is because the side of the vehicle provides less protection.

● If a driver is wearing a seatbelt and the vehicle is struck head-on or from behind, this may result in a whiplash injury, with strained muscles and sprained ligaments in the neck. There may also be bruising due to seatbelt restraint.
● If a victim dives into the shallow end of a swimming pool and hits his head, he is likely to sustain a neck injury.
● If a victim is thrown from a horse at speed and hits his head, he is likely to also have a neck injury.

Carrying out a head-to-toe survey

It is important to examine a victim from head to toe to assess the seriousness of her injuries. Signs and symptoms may change while you are looking after a victim. In addition, monitor her vital signs—level of response, pulse, and breathing (pp.20–1)—regularly. Look for clues, listen to what she says, feel for anything abnormal, and smell for anything unusual. Work along the body carefully, while talking reassuringly to the victim to calm her. Ask any questions that could be relevant to her condition.

1 Look for general signs and symptoms

● Ask the victim if she feels any pain and, if so, where.
● Feel her skin—it may be cold, clammy, hot, or sweaty.
● Watch her skin for blueness (cyanosis), especially around the lips.

● Check her breathing—it may be rapid, slow, shallow, or labored.
● Feel her pulse—it may be fast, slow, weak, or erratic.
● Watch the victim's level of response—she may be drowsy, confused, or anxious.

2 Examine head and neck

● Run your hands carefully over the victim's head. If you suspect a neck injury, be careful not to move the head. Feel for signs of any blood, swelling, or a depression in the skull—these are all signs of a skull fracture.
● Speak clearly into each ear and watch for the response.
● Look for any blood or a yellowish fluid coming from either ear or from the nose —these are signs of a skull fracture.
● Look for bleeding, bruising, swelling, or a foreign object in the eye. Ask if the victim can see clearly.

● Look to see if the victim's pupils are equal in size and constrict in response to light. If they are unequal in size, this could indicate cerebral compression.
● Look for bleeding, bruising, or swelling around the mouth.
● Detect any unpleasant odors on the breath by smelling near to the mouth.
● Loosen clothing at the neck and look for a hole (stoma) in the windpipe left by a surgical operation, or a medical warning necklace.
● Ask the victim if she has any neck pain. Feel the collarbones for deformity.

Looking for external clues

If a victim is unable to cooperate, look for the following clues:
● Objects that may have caused injury.
● Objects that may indicate the problem, such as used needles and syringes, alcohol bottles, or pots of glue.
● Medicines that may indicate the medical condition of the victim.
● An inhaler that may indicate asthma.

● An autoinjector that may indicate a risk of anaphylactic shock.
● A warning bracelet that gives a phone number to ring for information about the victim's medical history.
● A card that indicates a history of allergy, diabetes, or epilepsy.
● A special bracelet, necklace, card, or medallion carrying medical information.

3 Check chest and abdomen

- Look for any wounds to the chest, or abnormal movement.
- Ask the victim to take a deep breath and look to see if her chest expands evenly and equally on both sides—if not, this may indicate a chest injury.
- Listen for coughing or wheezing, as this may indicate asthma.
- Feel the ribcage for swelling, deformity, or tenderness.
- Look for wounds, bruising, or swelling of the abdomen.
- Feel for any tenderness or rigidity of the muscles—signs of an internal injury.

- Look at the clothing for signs of incontinence or bleeding from orifices.
- Feel the pelvis for any deformity.

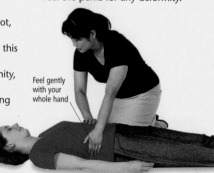

Feel gently with your whole hand

4 Assess whether there is back pain

- If the victim complains of severe back pain or difficulty moving the limbs, suspect a back injury and do not move the victim.

- Ask about numbness or tingling.
- If the victim has no sign of injury, ask if there is a previous history of back pain.

5 Look at arms and hands

- Look for any bleeding, bruising, swelling, or deformity.
- Ask the victim to move her arms at the different joints.
- Look for any needle marks or a medical warning device.
- Check the color of the fingers— if they are blue, this may indicate a problem with blood circulation or an injury caused by cold.

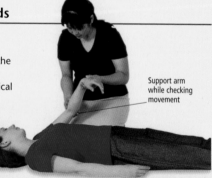

Support arm while checking movement

6 Check legs and feet

- Look for any bleeding, bruising, swelling, or deformity.
- Ask the victim to move the legs at the different joints.

- Check the color of her feet and toes —if they are blue, this could indicate a problem with blood circulation or an injury caused by cold.

Monitoring vital signs

While you are waiting for the EMS, it is important to keep monitoring the victim's level of response, pulse, and breathing. These vital signs will help you assess whether his condition is stable, worsening, or improving, or whether there are any specific problems. You may also need to check his body temperature. Write down your findings and the intervals between each assessment and give the information to medical staff or the emergency services.

Checking level of response

To help you assess a victim's level of consciousness, use the AVPU code. Follow this code at regular intervals, so that you can check whether the victim's condition is improving or deteriorating.

● A—Is the victim **Alert** and responding to you normally? This means that he is fully conscious.

● V—Does the victim respond to your **Voice**, answer simple questions, and obey simple commands?
● P—Does the victim respond to **Pain**?
● U—Is the victim **Unresponsive** to everything? This means that he is unconscious. Call 911 or local EMS and be ready to begin resuscitation (pp.36–52).

Checking pulse

● The normal pulse rate in adults is 60–80 beats per minute. In very fit young adults the pulse is slower and in children it is much faster—up to 140 beats per minute.
● Feel a victim's pulse at the neck (carotid pulse) or at the wrist (radial pulse). In infants, the easiest pulse to find is the brachial pulse in the upper arm.

● When checking a victim's pulse, use your fingers rather than your thumb (which has its own pulse) and press lightly downward in order to feel the beat.
● Using a watch, monitor and write down the following details: rate (the number of beats per minute); strength (whether the pulse is strong or weak); rhythm (whether the pulse is regular or irregular).

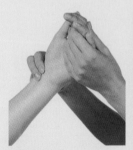

Radial pulse
Place two or three fingers just below the wrist creases at the base of the thumb. Use the pads of the fingers to improve sensitivity.

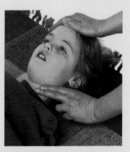

Carotid pulse
Place two fingers on the side of the victim's neck, in the hollow between the windpipe and the large neck muscle.

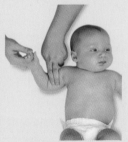

Brachial pulse
Place two fingers on the inner side of an infant's upper arm midway between the shoulder and elbow. Use the pads of the fingers to improve sensitivity.

Checking breathing rate

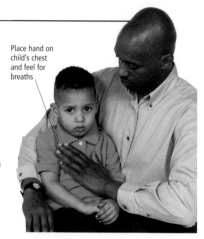

- The normal breathing rate in adults is 12–16 breaths and in young children 20–30 breaths per minute.

Place hand on child's chest and feel for breaths

- Listen to the victim's breaths, watch his chest rise and fall, and count the number of breaths in one minute.
- For young children, put your hand on the chest and feel for breathing.
- Listen carefully for any breathing difficulties or unusual noises.
- Using a watch, monitor and write down the following details: rate (number of breaths per minute); depth (deep or shallow breaths); quality (easy, difficult, or painful breaths); noise (quiet or noisy breathing).

Measuring temperature

- Normal body temperature is around 98.6°F (37°C). A high temperature is usually caused by infection; a low temperature (see Hypothermia p.86) may result from exposure to cold and/or wet weather conditions.
- To obtain an accurate temperature reading use a thermometer.
- There are several types of thermometer, including digital, forehead, and aural. Whichever type you have, make sure you know how to use it.
- A digital thermometer can be used under the tongue or in the armpit. Leave it in place for about 30 seconds until it "beeps"; then read the display.
- A forehead thermometer is useful for measuring temperature in a young child. Hold the small, heat-sensitive strip against the forehead for about 30 seconds and its color will change to indicate the temperature.
- An ear sensor, or aural thermometer, is useful for a child. Place its tip inside the ear to get a reading within one second.

WARNING

▶ Never put a digital thermometer in the mouth of a child under the age of seven. There is a risk that he or she may bite on it and break it.

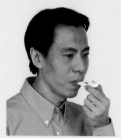

Digital thermometer

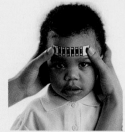

Forehead thermometer

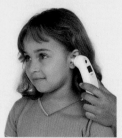

Aural thermometer

First-aid materials

Keep an easily identifiable first-aid kit in a safe, accessible place at home. There should also be one in the family car. The kit should be kept under a seat or in the trunk—never on the back shelf as it may fly off and cause an injury if the brakes are applied suddenly. You can buy a first-aid kit or assemble items yourself and store them in a clean, waterproof container. Dressings and bandages form the basis of a home first-aid kit, but there are a few useful extras. Check all the kit regularly; replace any out-of-date items.

Bandages

Small crepe bandage

Roller bandages
These are used to secure dressings and support injured limbs (p.26).

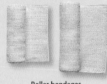

Roller bandages, small and large

Folded cloth bandage

Triangular bandages
Made of cloth or strong paper, these bandages are used to secure dressings (p.27) and to make slings (pp.28–9).

Folded paper bandage

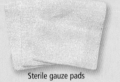

Sterile gauze pads

Gauze pads
Sterile gauze pads are versatile and can be used as padding under bandages, as dressings, or as swabs to clean around wounds.

Clear and fabric tape   Bandage clip   Safety pins

Tapes, clips, and pins
Adhesive tapes, bandage clips, and safety pins are all useful for securing the ends of bandages. Some bandages come with a clip attached.

Tying a square knot

Always use a square knot to secure a bandage or sling because it will not slip and it is also easy to undo. Since the knot lies flat against the victim, it is more comfortable. Follow the sequence below for tying a square knot.

● Hold one end of the bandage in each hand. Take the right end of the bandage over the left.

● Pass what is now the left end under and through the gap.

● Take what is now the right end over the left. Pass it through the gap and pull the knot tight to secure it.

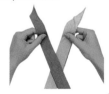

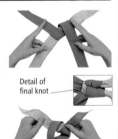

Detail of final knot

Dressings and adhesive bandages

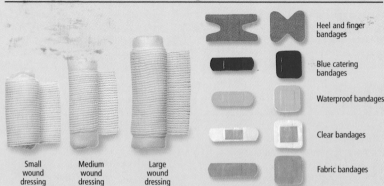

Small wound dressing

Medium wound dressing

Large wound dressing

Heel and finger bandages

Blue catering bandages

Waterproof bandages

Clear bandages

Fabric bandages

Sterile wound dressings
These dressings are sealed and come with an attached bandage, and in various sizes. They are placed on wounds to help control bleeding and prevent infection.

Assorted adhesive bandages
These bandages, made of fabric or waterproof plastic, are used to cover small cuts and abrasions. People who work with food have to use blue adhesive bandages.

Useful additions to a first-aid kit

Plastic face mask

Wound cleansing wipes

Disposable gloves

Scissors   Tweezers   Notepad and pencil

For protection
Disposable gloves should be worn whenever you come into contact with body fluids, such as blood. A face mask placed over a victim's mouth will protect you and the victim from infections when giving rescue breaths. Use wound cleansing wipes to clean the skin around wounds and to clean your hands if you have no soap and water.

Household items
There are a few household items that are useful to keep in a first-aid kit, such as scissors, tweezers, and a notepad and pencil or pen.

Foil survival bag

Plastic survival bag

Blanket

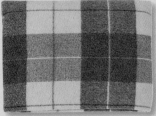

Warning triangle

For outdoors
Keep a flashlight, blanket, and a survival bag with a camping or car first-aid kit. Store a warning triangle in the trunk for placing at the site of a vehicle incident.

Sterile wound dressings

These absorbent gauze pads have been sterilized and individually sealed in protective wrapping. As soon as the protective wrapping is taken off, the dressing is no longer sterile. Make sure the dressing pad is large enough to extend beyond the edges of the wound. If any blood shows through after the dressing is secure, do not remove the dressing, but place another one on top. If blood seeps through the second dressing, remove both dressings and start again. If the dressing does not have a bandage attached, place the pad over the injury, and secure it with a separate bandage.

1 Unroll dressing

- Put on disposable gloves, if available.
- Unwrap the dressing and unroll the short end of the bandage until the end of the dressing pad is visible.
- Holding the bandage, open the pad next to the wound and place on the wound.

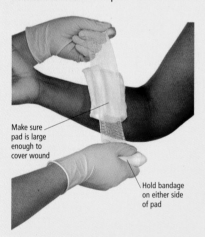

Make sure pad is large enough to cover wound

Hold bandage on either side of pad

2 Bandage over pad

- Hold the sterile pad in place on the injury and use the long end of the roller bandage to secure the pad by winding it around the affected body part.
- Make sure the bandage covers the whole of the pad.

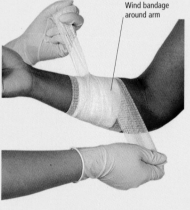

Wind bandage around arm

IMPORTANT
▶ Do not slide the pad onto the wound. Position it carefully over the wound.
▶ Do not touch the gauze side of the pad.

3 Secure bandage

- Tie the ends of the bandages in a square knot (p.22) over the pad.
- Check the circulation in the hand (p.26). If the bandage is too tight, loosen it and reapply.

Adhesive bandage

These bandages are used to cover small cuts and abrasions. Ask the victim if he is allergic to the adhesive before applying one. If he is, use a sterile dressing instead.

1 Open adhesive bandage pack

● Wash your hands and then open the sterile pack.

2 Put adhesive bandage on wound

● Taking care not to touch the pad in the center, gently pull back the plastic covers until the bandage pad is exposed.
● Place the bandage pad on the wound and pull the plastic covers further back until the dressing is secured in place.

Pull back plastic covers

Emergency dressings

If you do not have sterile wound dressings or adhesive bandage, you can use any piece of clean, nonfluffy material, such as a handkerchief.
● Wash your hands, hold the material by the corners, and let it fall open.
● Fold the material to the desired size so what was the inside surface, and probably cleaner, is now on the outside.
● Holding the material at the edges, place it over the wound and secure in place with a bandage, tape, or a scarf.
● If you have neither bandages nor material, cover the wound with a clean plastic bag or any clean item found in the kitchen, such as kitchen towel or plastic wrap.

Cold compresses

These are used to reduce bruising and swelling, which helps relieve pain. Apply for 10 minutes and then reassess the injury. You should reapply the cold compress at 10-minute intervals for up to 30 minutes, if necessary.

1 Wet a cloth

● Soak a face cloth, thin towel, or similar piece of material in cold water, then wring it out until it stops dripping.

2 Position pad over injury

● Fold the cloth to the required size and place it over the injury. If possible, replace the pad every 10 minutes, or cool it by dripping cold water onto it.

Using an ice pack

A plastic bag containing ice cubes or a bag of frozen peas or corn makes a very effective cold compress.
● Fill a plastic bag half- to two-thirds full of ice cubes.
● Squeeze the air out of the bag and seal it.

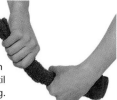

● Wrap the bag in a thin towel and place it over the victim's injury. Apply for 10 minutes and replace as necessary.

IMPORTANT
▶ Do not put ice directly onto the skin because it will burn.

Roller bandages

Use a roller bandage to support muscle or joint injuries, secure dressings, or to apply pressure to control bleeding. Once the bandage is secured, check the circulation in the fingers or toes beyond the bandage by pressing the skin until it turns pale and watching for color to return. If the color does not return, loosen the bandage.

1 Bandage around limb

- Place the end of the bandage on the limb and make a firm, straight turn to secure the bandage. Keep the injured part supported as you do so.

2 Work up limb

- Working up the limb, make a series of spiral turns with the bandage, allowing each successive turn to cover two-thirds of the previous one.

3 Secure bandage

- Finish winding with a straight turn.
- Secure the end with a safety pin, bandage clip, or tape. Alternatively, tuck in the remaining bandage.

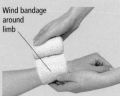
Wind bandage around limb

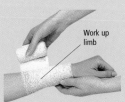
Work up limb

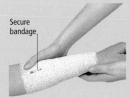
Secure bandage

Bandaging an ankle or hand

To support an ankle or hand injury, you need to adapt the bandaging technique. Extend the bandage well beyond the injury so that pressure is applied over the entire injured area. When bandaging a hand, start at the wrist and leave the thumb free.

1 Bandage around ankle

- Wind the bandage around the ankle and take it diagonally across the foot.
- Bring the bandage under the ball of the foot to the base of the big toe.

2 Bandage across foot

- Pass the bandage across the top of the victim's foot and back around the ankle.
- Make another straight turn around the ankle.

3 Secure bandage

- Continue figure-of-eight turns around the foot and ankle until they are covered.
- Make a final turn around the ankle and secure at the ankle as described above.

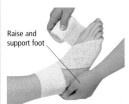
Raise and support foot

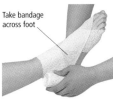
Take bandage across foot

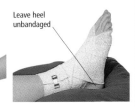
Leave heel unbandaged

Triangular bandages

Use a triangular bandage to make slings and to secure injured limbs. Although they are usually made from unbleached calico, you can make one yourself from similar material about 3ft (1m) square cut diagonally in half. The bandage can be folded in two ways: broad-fold and narrow-fold, or cravat. A broad-fold bandage is used mainly to immobilize and support a limb; a cravat bandage is most commonly used to immobilize feet and ankles.

Point

Base

Open triangular bandage

1 Broad-fold bandage

● Lay the bandage on a flat, clean surface, and fold the point of the triangular bandage to the base.
● Fold the bandage in half again.

Broad-fold bandage

2 Cravat bandage

● Fold a broad-fold bandage in half along its length.

Cravat bandage

Cover bandages

A triangular bandage can also be used to hold a light dressing in place, especially on a hand or foot—but it is not suitable for controlling bleeding.

1 Fold bandage over hand

● Place the victim's hand on the bandage.
● Bring the point of the bandage over the hand onto the forearm.

Fold point of bandage over hand

2 Wrap bandage around hand

● Pass the two ends of the triangular bandage around the wrist, crossing over the hand in opposite directions.

Do not wrap bandage too tightly

3 Tie ends together

● Tie the two ends together in a square knot (p.22) above the point of the bandage.
● Gently pull the point of the bandage down to tighten and secure the bandage over the dressing.

Knot lies flat on limb

Detail of knot

4 Secure bandage

● Lift the point of the bandage over the square knot. Tuck in the point or secure it over the square knot with a safety pin.

Cover knot with point of bandage

Detail of tuck

Arm sling

Use an arm sling to support an injured upper arm, forearm, or wrist and to immobilize an arm if there is a chest injury. Like the elevation sling (opposite), an arm sling should be used only if the victim is able to bend his elbow.

You will need
▶ Triangular bandage
▶ Safety pin

IMPORTANT
▶ Keep the injured arm well supported until the sling is secure and supports the arm itself.

1 Support injured arm

● Sit the victim down and ask him to support the injured arm with his other arm.
● Slide one end of a triangular bandage through the hollow under his elbow.
● Pull the upper end until it rests by the collarbone on the side of the injury.

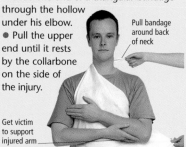

Pull bandage around back of neck

Get victim to support injured arm

2 Secure sling

● Bring the lower end of the bandage up over the forearm so that it supports the injured arm.
● Tie a square knot (p.22) in the hollow above the collarbone on the injured side.
● Tuck the ends of the bandage under the square knot.

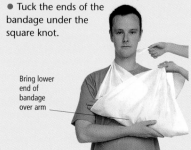

Bring lower end of bandage over arm

3 Pin bandage at elbow

● Tuck the excess bandage behind the elbow and secure the point with either a safety pin (below) or a twist (opposite).

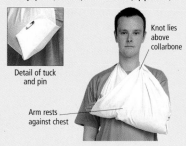

Detail of tuck and pin

Knot lies above collarbone

Arm rests against chest

Improvising an arm sling

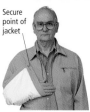

Secure point of jacket

● For a zip-up jacket, turn the open jacket up over the arm and attach it to the top of the jacket with a safety pin.

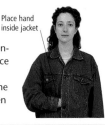

Place hand inside jacket

● For a button-up jacket, place the victim's hand inside the jacket between its fastenings.

Elevation sling

Use this type of sling to support the arm in a raised position when a hand or forearm is injured and bleeding needs to be controlled, to support a broken hand, to reduce swelling, and to support the arm in the event of a broken collarbone or rib.

You will need
▶ Triangular bandage
▶ Safety pin

IMPORTANT
▶ Keep the injured arm well supported until the sling is secure and supports the arm itself.

1 Support injured arm

● Sit the victim down and ask her to support her arm across the chest so that the fingers reach the opposite shoulder.

Support arm at elbow

2 Position bandage

● Lay a triangular bandage over her arm with one end over the shoulder, making sure the point is past the elbow.

Lay bandage across arm

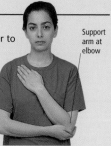

Longest edge of bandage

3 Tuck in bandage

● Tuck the base of the bandage under the victim's forearm and elbow.
● Take the lower end of the bandage around the victim's back and up towards the other shoulder.

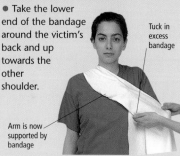

Tuck in excess bandage

Arm is now supported by bandage

4 Secure sling

● Tie both ends of the bandage together in the hollow above the collarbone using a square knot (p.22).
● Secure the point of the bandage with a safety pin (opposite). If you do not have a pin, twist the point of the bandage and tuck it in above the elbow (below).
● Check the circulation in the thumb (p.26).

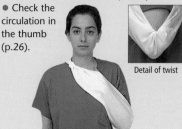

Detail of twist

Improvising an elevation sling

● A turned-up jumper can be used to support an arm.

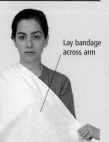

Secure hand against shoulder

Test yourself

Now that you have read and studied the chapter on first-aid principles, see if you can answer the questions below. After completing the questions, check your answers against the correct ones on page 144.

1 What should you do first when arriving at the scene of an incident?
....
....

2 What should you do if there is a major incident such as a fire?
....
....

3 When dealing with several victims at the same time, which ones should you tend to first?
....
....

4 What should you wear if you are likely to come into contact with body fluids such as blood?
....

5 What is a sharp object container?
....
....

6 How do you get in touch with the emergency services?
....
....

7 When checking level of response, what does AVPU stand for?
A..
V..
P..
U..

8 Where on the body can you feel a pulse?
....
....
....

9 Which of the following are basic items for a first-aid kit?
a Sterile wound dressings.................... ☐
b Blanket .... ☐
c Triangular bandage .... ☐
d Adhesive bandages .... ☐
e Scissors.. ☐
f Safety pins.. ☐

10 Why is a square knot a good way to secure a bandage?
....
....

11 Why should you not put ice directly onto the skin?
....
....

12 How do you check that a bandage on a hand or foot is not too tight?
....
....

13 For what reasons would you use an arm sling and an elevation sling?
Arm sling..
....
....

Elevation sling ....
....
....
....
....

2 Life-saving techniques

To stay alive, the body needs a continuous supply of oxygen. This chapter shows you how to maintain the supply of oxygen for a victim who is not breathing. It provides an up-to-date guide to the life-saving techniques used to treat victims who are unconscious or choking.

Easy-to-understand anatomical information explains how the breathing and blood circulation systems work, to help you understand why the resuscitation techniques are effective. The methods used vary for adults, children, and infants so there are separate life-saving sequences for each.

This chapter includes instructions for using an automated external defibrillator (AED)—also known as a defibrillator—a machine that can be used to treat a victim whose heart has stopped beating.

Once you have studied this chapter, use the questionnaire on page 56 to test your knowledge and understanding of the procedures described here.

Contents

Dealing with unconsciousness

If a victim is unconscious, her airway can become blocked so she may stop breathing. Your priority is to open the airway to get air to her lungs so that oxygen can reach her brain and other vital organs. All parts of the body, especially the brain, need oxygen to function and remain alive. When air is breathed in and drawn into the lungs, oxygen in the air passes into the blood and is carried to all parts of the body (p.34). If the victim is not breathing and the heart is not beating (cardiac arrest), you need to give cardiopulmonary resuscitation (CPR)—a combination of rescue breaths and chest compressions. CPR sequences for adults, children, and infants can be found on pages 36–52.

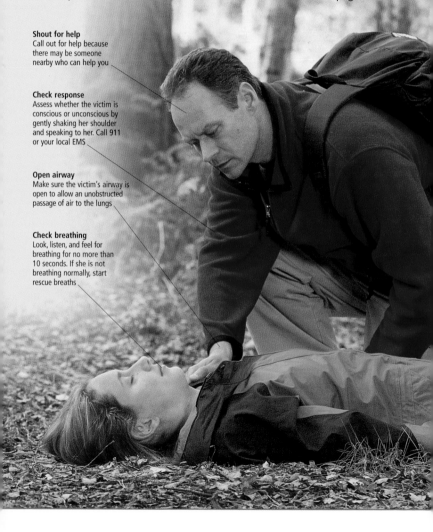

Shout for help
Call out for help because there may be someone nearby who can help you

Check response
Assess whether the victim is conscious or unconscious by gently shaking her shoulder and speaking to her. Call 911 or your local EMS

Open airway
Make sure the victim's airway is open to allow an unobstructed passage of air to the lungs

Check breathing
Look, listen, and feel for breathing for no more than 10 seconds. If she is not breathing normally, start rescue breaths

What you should do

IMPORTANT
▶ For an adult or child who is not breathing, a machine called an automated external defibrillator, or defibrillator, can be used to try to restart the heart. Ask a bystander to find one if possible.

WARNING
▶ Make sure there is no danger to you or the victim as you approach the scene.

Your aims
▶ Check victim's response
▶ Establish and maintain an open airway
▶ Check for breathing and give CPR—rescue breaths followed by chest compressions—if necessary

IMPORTANT
▶ If a defibrillator is available, have it brought to the scene. Attach it immediately and follow instructions (pp.44–5).

1 Check response

● Speak to the victim loudly and clearly.
● Shake the victim's shoulder gently.
● If there is no response, shout for help.

2 Call 911 or local EMS

● Ideally send a helper to make the call and bring a defibrillator.

3 Open airway

● Place one hand on the forehead and tilt the head.
● Place your other hand on the point of the chin and lift the victim's chin.

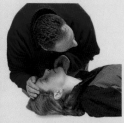

4 Check breathing

● Look, listen, and feel for normal breathing for no more than 10 seconds.

5 Start rescue breathing

● If the victim is not breathing give her two rescue breaths.

6 Begin chest compressions

● Follow rescue breaths with 30 chest compressions.
● Continue alternating 30 compresssions with two rescue breaths (CPR) until help arrives and takes over, the victim starts to breathe normally, or you are too tired to continue.

7 Put in recovery position

● If the victim is breathing or resumes normal breathing, place her in the recovery position.

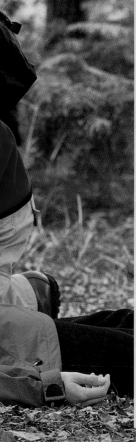

Breathing and blood circulation

Oxygen is essential to life—every cell in the body needs it to be able to function. If deprived of oxygen for any length of time, the cells die—those in the brain survive only minutes without an adequate supply. Oxygen is taken in when we breathe in via the airway and the lungs (respiratory system). It is then transported around the body by the heart and blood vessels (circulatory system).

How the body gets oxygen

As we breathe in, muscles in the chest wall and diaphragm contract, the chest cavity enlarges, and air containing oxygen enters the body through the mouth and nose and passes into the windpipe, or airway. The airway divides into two smaller tubes (bronchi), one for each lung. In the lungs, the bronchi divide into smaller tubes called bronchioles that end in microscopic air sacs (alveoli). Oxygen from the air we breathe in passes through the walls of these air sacs into small blood vessels (capillaries), where it is picked up by the blood. The oxygen-rich blood is then carried to the heart and pumped around the body. When we breathe out, the muscles in the chest wall and diaphragm relax, the chest cavity contracts, and the lungs shrink, sending used air up the airway and out of the body.

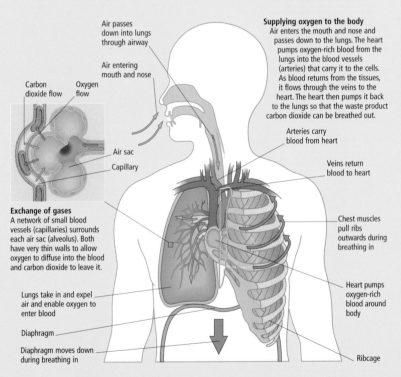

Air passes
down into lungs
through airway

Air entering
mouth and nose

Carbon   Oxygen
dioxide flow   flow

Air sac

Capillary

Exchange of gases
A network of small blood
vessels (capillaries) surrounds
each air sac (alveolus). Both
have very thin walls to allow
oxygen to diffuse into the blood
and carbon dioxide to leave it.

Lungs take in and expel
air and enable oxygen to
enter blood

Diaphragm

Diaphragm moves down
during breathing in

Supplying oxygen to the body
Air enters the mouth and nose and
passes down to the lungs. The heart
pumps oxygen-rich blood from the
lungs into the blood vessels
(arteries) that carry it to the cells.
As blood returns from the tissues,
it flows through the veins to the
heart. The heart then pumps it back
to the lungs so that the waste product
carbon dioxide can be breathed out.

Arteries carry
blood from heart

Veins return
blood to heart

Chest muscles
pull ribs
outwards during
breathing in

Heart pumps
oxygen-rich
blood around
body

Ribcage

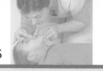
How resuscitation works

With an unconscious victim, breathing and circulation may not function properly, so the body's cells are starved of oxygen. The possibility of recovery decreases rapidly, within a few minutes. By using cardiopulmonary resuscitation (CPR), which involves keeping the victim's airway open, giving him rescue breaths to imitate breathing and chest compressions to keep blood circulating, you can supply oxygen to the victim until emergency aid arrives. This is easy to remember as the ABC of resuscitation—A is for airway, B for breathing, and C for chest compressions. A machine called a defibrillator can be used to restart the heart (p.44).

Agonal breathing is common in the first few minutes after a heart stops (cardiac arrest). It is usually in the form of infrequent short gasps for breath. If present it should not be mistaken for normal breathing and you should start CPR without hesitation.

Opening the airway

Loss of muscle control in an unconscious victim, can cause the tongue to fall back and block the airway. When this happens, breathing becomes difficult and noisy, or impossible. Tilting the head back and lifting the chin lifts the tongue, allowing the victim to breathe.

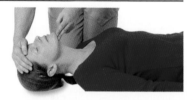

Breathing for a victim

The air that we breathe out contains about 16 percent oxygen, which is five percent less than in the air that we breathe in. By giving rescue breaths, you can force air into the victim's airway. This air reaches the air sacs (alveoli) in the lungs and oxygen is then transferred to the small blood vessels within the lungs.

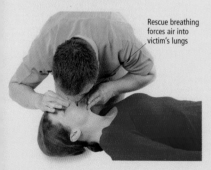

Rescue breathing forces air into victim's lungs

Maintaining circulation

If the heart stops beating, oxygenated blood does not circulate around the body and oxygen cannot reach the vital organs, such as the brain. Chest compressions act as a mechanical aid to get some blood flowing around the body. Pushing vertically down on the center of the chest squeezes the chest and heart, forcing blood around the body. As pressure is released, the chest rises, allowing replacement blood to flow into the chest.

Pushing down on chest using correct technique can keep blood circulating

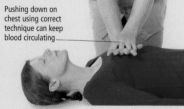

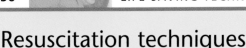

Resuscitation techniques

This section sets out the life-saving measures needed to ensure that an adequate supply of oxygen reaches the vital organs, such as the brain, heart, and kidneys, in an unconscious victim. It is divided into three main parts: for adults, for children aged one to eight, and for infants (children under one year old). Each part outlines initial checks, the recovery position, and then describes the techniques—chest compressions and rescue breathing (cardiopulmonary resuscitation or CPR)—that you need to help restore and maintain a victim's breathing and circulation.

Resuscitation plan

This is a summary of the different stages that are needed to resuscitate an unconscious adult, child, or infant. Check for danger before approaching the victim (p.16). You can perform all of the stages of resuscitation kneeling next to the victim's head or chest.

CHECK RESPONSE
(p.37 adults; p.46 children; p.50 infants)
● Shout and shake (adults) or tap (children) shoulder
● Infants: shout and tap sole of foot
● **Is there a response from the victim?**
| YES →

● Treat any injuries
● Adults and children: leave in position found and get medical help if necessary
● Infants: take with you to summon help if necessary
● Call 911 or local EMS if necessary

NO ↓

✚ CALL 911 OR LOCAL EMS
Get a helper to do this if possible and ask him or her to bring a defibrillator if available

● Check for life-threatening injuries
● Place victim in recovery position (p.38 adults; p.47 children; p.51 infants)

CHECK BREATHING
(p.37 adults; p.46 children; p.50 infants)
● Tilt head back
● Lift up chin to hold airway open
● Look, listen, and feel for breath for up to 10 seconds
● **Is victim breathing normally?**
| YES →

NO ↓

BEGIN RESCUE BREATHING
(p.40 adults; p.48 children; p.51 infants)
● Give two rescue breaths at a rate on one breath per second

↓

BEGIN CHEST COMPRESSIONS
(p.42 adults; p.49 children; p.52 infants)
● Give 30 chest compressions at a rate of 100 compressions per minute
● Repeat two more rescue breaths
● Continue alternating chest compressions and rescue breaths 30:2 (cardiopulmonary resuscitation/CPR) until emergency help arrives, the victim starts to breathe normally, or you are too exhausted to keep going

WARNING
▶ If you are alone and an adult victim is not breathing normally, call 911 or local EMS immediately then continue resuscitation.
▶ If you are alone and the victim is a child or infant, give CPR for two minutes (about 5 cycles) before calling the emergency services.

IMPORTANT
▶ If you are familiar only with the adult sequence for CPR you may use this on a child, using one hand only for a small child.

ADULT LIFE-SAVING SEQUENCE

Check response

⬇

If victim does not respond,

⬇

✚ CALL 911 OR LOCAL EMS

⬇

Check breathing

⬇

If victim is breathing normally, place in recovery position

OR

If victim is not breathing, or is not breathing normally

⬇

Begin rescue breathing

⬇

Begin chest compressions

⬇

Continue chest compressions and rescue breaths (CPR)

Check response (adult)

If you discover a collapsed victim, you need to decide if he is conscious or unconscious. Follow the instructions below for an adult victim.

Check consciousness

● Gently shake the victim's shoulders and ask "What has happened?" or give a command such as "Open your eyes."

If the victim responds,

● leave her in the position in which you found her and get help if necessary. Treat any injuries.

If the victim does not respond,

● shout for help.

✚ **CALL 911 OR LOCAL EMS**

send a helper, if available, or make the call yourself.

Check breathing (adult)

If the victim is unconscious, you should use the head tilt and chin lift to open her airway, then check breathing.

1 Open airway

● Place one hand on the victim's forehead and gently tilt her head back.
● Lift the chin with the index and middle fingers of your other hand.

2 Look, listen, and feel for breathing

● Look along the chest for movement, listen for breathing, and feel for breath on your cheek for no more than 10 seconds.

If the victim is breathing normally,

● Check for life-threatening injuries.
● Place her in the recovery position (overleaf).

If the victim is not breathing or is not breathing normally,

● Begin rescue breathing (p.40).

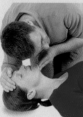

ADULT LIFE-SAVING SEQUENCE

Check response

If victim does not respond,

✚ CALL 911 OR LOCAL EMS

Check breathing

If victim is breathing normally, place in **recovery position**

OR

If victim is not breathing, or is not breathing normally

Begin rescue breathing

Begin chest compressions

Continue chest compressions and rescue breaths (CPR)

Recovery position (adult)

If the victim is unconscious but breathing normally, place her in the recovery position. Follow the instructions below if she is lying on her back. If she is already lying on her side, do not follow entire sequence, but make sure she is in a stable position and cannot roll onto her back.

1 Remove glasses and bulky objects from pockets

● Straighten the victim's legs.
● Remove glasses if she is wearing them, and any bulky items, such as a cell phone or keys, from her pockets.

2 Move arm nearest to you

● Place the arm nearest to you at a right angle to the victim's body, with the palm facing up.

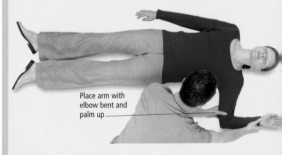

Place arm with elbow bent and palm up

3 Move other arm and raise leg

● Bring the arm furthest from you across the victim's chest and hold her hand, palm outwards, against the cheek nearest to you.
● With your other hand, get hold of the knee furthest from you and pull the leg up until the foot is flat on the floor.

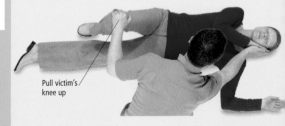

Pull victim's knee up

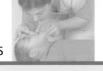

4 Pull knee towards you

- With one hand, keep the victim's hand pressed against her cheek to support the head.
- With your other hand, pull the leg towards you, rolling the victim onto her side.

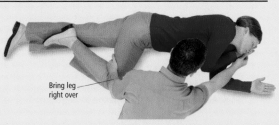

Bring leg right over

5 Position leg at right angle

- Pull the victim's top leg up at a right angle to the body, so that both the hip and knee are bent at right angles.

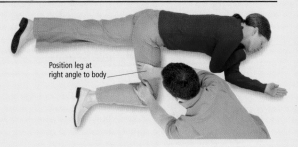

Position leg at right angle to body

6 Keep airway open

- Make sure the victim's airway remains open.
- If the hand under her cheek has moved, put it back into position to help keep the head tilted.

7 Monitor victim

- Monitor and record the victim's vital signs—level of response, pulse, and breathing (pp.20–1)— regularly until help arrives.

For a suspected spinal injury

If you suspect a victim has a spinal injury, place her in the recovery position if you are unable to keep her airway open using the jaw-thrust method (p.111) or if you are alone and have to leave her to get help. It is important to keep her neck and back straight while putting her in the recovery position.

- Extend one of the victims arm above her head, then roll her so that her head rests on the extended arm. Stabilize her legs as above.
- If there is one helper, one person holds the head steady as the other turns the victim.
- If there are two helpers available, one person holds the victim's head steady, one turns her, the third keeps the victim's back straight while she is being turned.

ADULT LIFE-SAVING SEQUENCE

Check response

If victim does
not respond,

✚ CALL 911 OR
LOCAL EMS

Check breathing

If victim is
breathing normally,
place in recovery
position

OR

If victim is not breathing,
or is not breathing
normally

Begin **rescue breathing**

Begin chest
compressions

Continue chest
compressions and rescue
breaths (CPR)

Rescue breathing (adult)

If an adult victim is not breathing normally, you will need
to begin rescue breaths immediately.

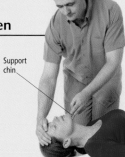

1 Keep airway open

● Make sure the victim's
head remains tilted back by
keeping one hand on her
forehead and supporting
her chin with the index and
middle fingers of your other
hand.

Support
chin

2 Begin rescue breaths

● Pinch the victim's nose.
● Take a normal (NOT deep)
breath, and then seal your lips
over the victim's mouth.
● Blow firmly and steadily
into the mouth for about
one second. If you are
sucessful you will see the
chest rise.
● If you cannot blow into her
mouth, close it and seal your
lips around her nose. After
each breath open her mouth
to allow the air to escape
from the lungs.

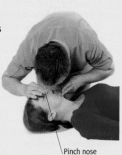

Pinch nose
with one hand

Using a face mask

A barrier device reduces
the risk of infection when
giving rescue breaths.
● Place the face mask over
the victim's face with the
filter over the mouth.
● Pinch his nose and
give rescue breaths
through the filter.

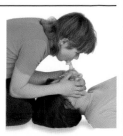

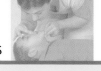

3 Repeat breath

- Lift your mouth away from the victim's mouth and look along her chest, watching it fall back. If the chest rises as you blow and falls when you remove your mouth, you have given a rescue breath.
- Give a second rescue breath.
- If the chest does not rise, check that her head is far enough back and that you have closed her nose completely. Check the mouth and remove any obvious obstruction.
- Make no more than two attempts at rescue breaths before beginning chest compressions. Do not stop to check victim's circulation.

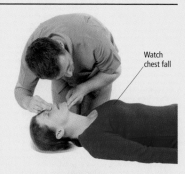

Watch chest fall

4 Begin chest compressions

- Give 30 chest compressions at a rate of 100 compressions per minute, see overleaf.
- Deliver cycles of 30 chest compressions followed by two rescue breaths.

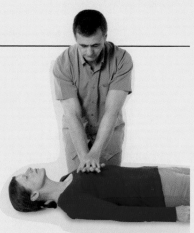

5 Put a breathing victim in recovery position

- If the victim begins to breathe normally, place her in the recovery position (p.38).
- Monitor and record her vital signs (pp.20–1) regularly until help arrives.

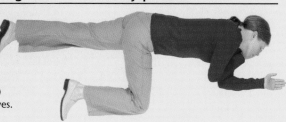

Chest compressions (adult)

Begin chest compressions immediately after giving rescue breaths, don't stop to check breathing or circulation. In most adult victims the heart will have stopped because of a heart (cardiac) problem, so a combination of rescue breaths and chest compressions is important to simulate blood circulation and breathing.

1 Place hand on center of chest

● Place the heel of one hand on the center of the victim's chest. This is the point where you will apply pressure. You can do this through clothing.

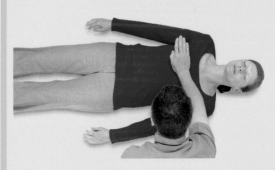

2 Cover hand

● Cover the first hand with your other hand and interlock your fingers.
● Make sure the fingers of both hands underneath are lifted clear of the victim's chest.
● Make sure you do not press on the ribs, the bottom tip of the breastbone, or the soft upper abdomen.

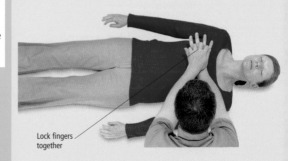

Lock fingers together

3 Give chest compressions

● Kneel up with your shoulders over the breastbone and your arms straight.
● Press down "hard and fast," one-third to one-half the depth of the chest.
● Release the pressure on the chest to let it recoil, or reexpand to its normal position, after each compression, but do not remove your hands.
● Give 30 chest compressions in total at a rate of 100 per minute. Use approximately equal compression and relaxation times.

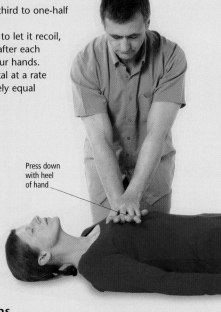

Press down with heel of hand

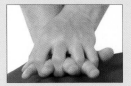

Detail of hands on chest

4 Repeat rescue breaths

● After chest compressions, repeat two rescue breaths (p.40).
● Continue cycles of 30 compressions to two rescue breaths until medical help arrives and takes over, the victim starts breathing normally, or you become too exhausted to continue.

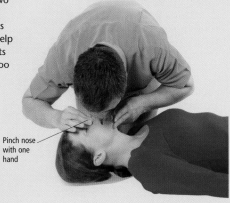

Pinch nose with one hand

IMPORTANT
▶ Limit interruptions in chest compressions—when you stop the blood flow stops. The early compressions are never as effective as the later ones.
▶ If you have a helper, swap every two minutes (after a set of 30 compressions) with as little disruption as possible to maintain good quality compressions.

Using a defibrillator

When a victim has a cardiac arrest, the heart stops beating so there is no circulation. A cardiac arrest may occur after a heart attack in which the normal heart rhythm is disturbed, causing a condition known as ventricular fibrillation. A machine known as an automated external defibrillator (AED), or defibrillator, can be used to try to reverse abnormal heart rhythm and restart a heart. Defibrillators can be found in many public places, including airports, railway stations, shopping centers, and offices, where staff are trained in their use. To use a defibrillator you must be trained and able to carry out cardiopulmonary resuscitation (CPR). In most cases when a defibrillator is called for, you will have already started CPR, continue while the defibrillator is prepared, give one shock then repeat CPR, see below and opposite.

1 Get defibrillator ready

- Switch on the defibrillator and take out the pads.

2 Remove victim's upper clothing

- Remove or cut through any clothing covering the chest and wipe away any sweat with a dry cloth.
- Shave the chest hair only if there is so much of it that it will stop the pads sticking to the skin.

3 Put pads on chest

- Attach the pads. Place one pad on the upper right side of the victim's chest, place the other one on the left side of the chest positioned so that its long axis is vertical.
- Stand clear and make sure no one is touching the victim because this will prevent the machine from making an accurate analysis.

Follow spoken or visual prompts of defibrillator

Position pads either side of heart

WARNING

▶ If at any time the victim starts breathing normally, place him in the recovery position (p.38), leaving the defibrillator attached.

▶ Do not use a defibrillator on an infant under the age of one year, or use a pediatric defibrillator on an adult.

4 Follow defibrillator prompts

- Follow the spoken or visual prompts given by the machine. It will tell you when to give a shock, and when to do CPR. If you need to give a shock, make sure nobody is touching the victim.
- Continue to follow the prompts until the emergency services arrive and take over from you.
- Do not remove the pads or switch off the defibrillator, even if the victim appears to have recovered.

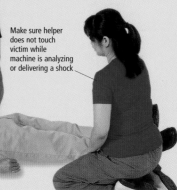

Make sure helper does not touch victim while machine is analyzing or delivering a shock

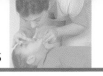
Sequence for using a defibrillator

When you use a defibrillator, it will give you a series of spoken and visual prompts (these vary from one machine to another). Once the pads are attached to a victim's chest, the defibrillator will analyze his heart rhythm. The chart below outlines the sequence for using the machine. All rescuers should give one shock followed immediately by CPR. Once all machines have been reprogrammed you will be advised to give a rhythm check after two minutes.

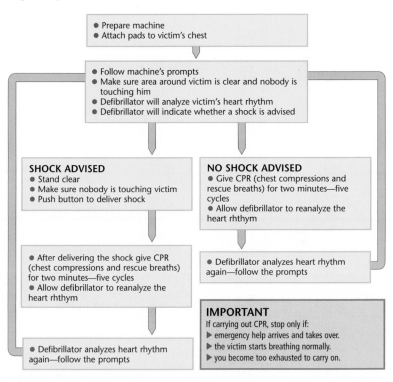

- Prepare machine
- Attach pads to victim's chest

- Follow machine's prompts
- Make sure area around victim is clear and nobody is touching him
- Defibrillator will analyze victim's heart rhythm
- Defibrillator will indicate whether a shock is advised

SHOCK ADVISED
- Stand clear
- Make sure nobody is touching victim
- Push button to deliver shock

NO SHOCK ADVISED
- Give CPR (chest compressions and rescue breaths) for two minutes—five cycles
- Allow defibrillator to reanalyze the heart rhthym

- After delivering the shock give CPR (chest compressions and rescue breaths) for two minutes—five cycles
- Allow defibrillator to reanalyze the heart rhthym

- Defibrillator analyzes heart rhythm again—follow the prompts

- Defibrillator analyzes heart rhythm again—follow the prompts

IMPORTANT
If carrying out CPR, stop only if:
▶ emergency help arrives and takes over.
▶ the victim starts breathing normally.
▶ you become too exhausted to carry on.

Pediatric defibrillators

Standard defibrillators can be used for children over the age of eight years. Pediatric defibrillators, or pediatric pads and a standard machine should be used on children over the age of one year if possible. If neither is available, then use a standard machine. Do not use a defibrillator on a infant aged under one year.

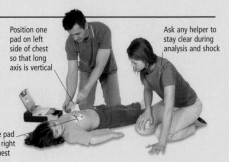

Position one pad on left side of chest so that long axis is vertical

Ask any helper to stay clear during analysis and shock

Place one pad on upper right side of chest

CHILD LIFE-SAVING SEQUENCE

Check response

If child does not respond,

Ask a helper to
✚ **CALL 911 OR LOCAL EMS**

Check breathing

If breathing, place in **recovery position**

OR

If not breathing normally,

Give two rescue breaths

Begin chest compressions and rescue breaths (CPR)

Repeat for two minutes and
✚ **CALL 911 OR LOCAL EMS**
if a call has not already been made

Continue CPR

Check response (child 1–8)

If a child has collapsed, you need to find out if he is conscious and breathing. Follow these instructions for a child aged one to eight years. See page 50 for an infant.

Check consciousness

● Call out the child's name, or give a command such as "Open your eyes", to try to provoke a response.
● Tap him on the shoulder.

WARNING
▶ Never shake a child to check if he is conscious or not.

If the child responds,
● leave him in the position in which you found him and get help if necessary. Treat any injuries.
If the child does not respond,
● shout for help and send a helper to
✚ **CALL 911 OR LOCAL EMS**
If you are on your own, open the airway and check breathing

Check breathing (child)

If the child is unconscious, open his airway, and check to see if he is breathing normally.

1 Open airway

● Place one hand on the child's forehead and gently tilt the head back.
● Lift the chin with the index and middle fingers of your other hand.
● Do not push on the soft part of the chin as it can block the airway.

2 Look, listen, and feel for breathing

● Look along the chest for movement, listen for breathing, and feel for breath on your cheek for no more than 10 seconds.
If the child is breathing normally,
● check for life-threatening injuries.
● Place him in the recovery position (opposite).
If the child is not breathing,
● begin rescue breathing (p.48).

Recovery position (child 1–8)

If a child aged between one year and eight years is unconscious and breathing, you should place her in the recovery position. If she is already lying on her side, you should make sure that she cannot roll onto her back as this may affect her breathing.

1 Straighten legs and position arm

- Kneel beside the child.
- Straighten her legs.
- Remove glasses and any bulky items from the pockets.
- Place the arm closest to you at a right angle to the child's body.

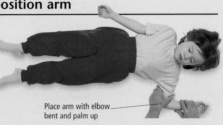

Place arm with elbow bent and palm up

2 Move other arm and raise leg

- Bring the child's far arm across her chest.
- Hold her hand, palm outwards, against her near cheek.
- With your other hand, grasp the knee furthest from you and pull the leg up until the foot is flat on the floor.

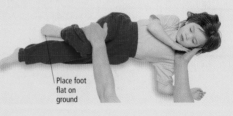

Place foot flat on ground

3 Roll child towards you

- With one hand, keep the child's hand pressed against her cheek to support her head.
- With the other hand, pull her far leg towards you, rolling her onto her side.
- Adjust the upper leg so that both the hip and the knee are bent at right angles.
- Tilt her head back to make sure her airway remains open.

✚ CALL 911 OR LOCAL EMS

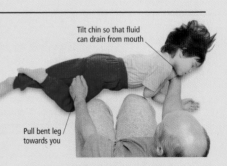

Tilt chin so that fluid can drain from mouth

Pull bent leg towards you

4 Monitor child

- Monitor and record the child's vital signs —level of response, pulse, and breathing (pp.20–1)—regularly until help arrives.

IMPORTANT
▶ If you think that the child might have damaged her neck or spine, follow the instructions given on page 39 for placing someone with a suspected spinal injury into the recovery position.

CHILD LIFE-SAVING SEQUENCE

Check response

If child does
not respond,

Ask a helper to
✚ **CALL 911 OR
LOCAL EMS**

Check breathing

If breathing, place in
recovery position

OR

If not breathing
normally,

**Give two rescue
breaths**

**Begin chest
compressions and
rescue breaths (CPR)**

Repeat for two minutes
and
✚ **CALL 911 OR
LOCAL EMS**
if a call has not already
been made

Continue CPR

Rescue breathing (child 1–8)

If a child is not breathing normally, start CPR a combination of rescue breaths (to get oxygen into the lungs) and chest compressions (to circulate the blood).

1 Keep airway open

● Make sure the head is tilted back by keeping one hand on his forehead and lift his chin by placing the index and middle fingers of your other hand on his chin.

2 Clear any obstructions from mouth

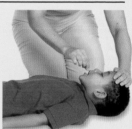

● Look in the child's mouth for obvious obstructions.
● Pick out anything you see with your thumb and forefinger.
● Do not do a fingersweep of his mouth.

3 Give rescue breaths

● Pinch the child's nose. Take a normal (not deep) breath, open your mouth, and seal your lips over the child's mouth.
● Blow firmly and steadily into the mouth for about one second, watch the chest rise.
● Give two rescue breaths.
● If the chest does not rise, check that his head is far enough back and that you have closed his nose completely.
● After two breaths (or attempts at breaths) begin chest compressions, opposite.

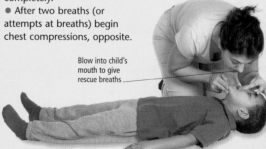

Blow into child's
mouth to give
rescue breaths

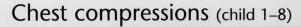

Chest compressions (child 1–8)

After two attempts at rescue breaths begin chest compressions. Do not stop to check circulation. If you are alone do CPR—rescue breaths and chest compressions—for two minutes (about five cycles) before stopping to call the emergency services.

1 Position hand on chest

- Place the heel of one hand on the center of the child's chest level with the nipple line. This is the point at which you press down on the chest.
- Take care not to press on the ribs, the lower tip of the breastbone, or the soft upper abdomen.

Press down straight with heel of hand, keeping fingers lifted

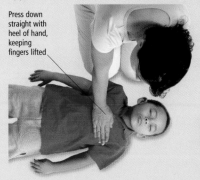

2 Give chest compressions

- Lean over the child, keeping your arm straight and keep your fingers lifted so you do not press down on to the ribs.
- Press down vertically on the breastbone with the heel of your hand, "push hard and push fast," about one-third to one-half of the depth of the chest.
- Release the pressure on the chest to let it come back up to its normal position, but do not remove your hands.
- Do this 30 times at a rate of 100 compressions per minute.

IMPORTANT
▶ If the child starts breathing normally, place him in the recovery position (p.47).

3 Give two rescue breaths

- After giving 30 chest compressions, tilt the child's head back, lift the chin, and repeat two rescue breaths (opposite).

Pinch nostrils together and give two rescue breaths

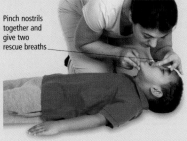

4 Alternate compressions with rescue breaths

- Carry on giving cycles of 30 chest compressions and two rescue breaths, maintaining the rate of 100 compressions per minute, for two minutes.

➕ **CALL 911 OR LOCAL EMS**
- Continue until help arrives and takes over, the child starts breathing, or you become too exhausted to continue.

For larger child or a small first aider

If you are small, or the child is large, give compressions with two hands as for an adult.
- Place one hand on the center of the child's chest as for an adult.
- Cover with your other hand and interlock your fingers, keeping your fingers raised.

INFANT LIFE-SAVING SEQUENCE

Check response

If infant does not respond,

Ask a helper to
✚ **CALL 911 OR LOCAL EMS**

Check breathing

If breathing, place in **recovery position**

OR

If not breathing normally,

Give two rescue breaths

Begin chest compressions and rescue breaths (CPR)

Repeat for two minutes and
✚ **CALL 911 OR LOCAL EMS**
if a call has not already been made

Continue CPR

Check response (infant)

This sequence is for an infant under the age of one year. It is easier to treat an infant if you place him on his back

Check consciousness

● Tap the sole of the infant's foot and call his name, if you know it.

If the infant responds,
● take him with you to get medical help if needed. Treat any injuries.

WARNING
▶ Never shake an infant to check if he is conscious.

If the infant does not respond,
● shout for help and send a helper to
✚ **CALL 911 OR LOCAL EMS**
If you are on your own, open the airway and check breathing.

Check breathing (infant)

If the infant is unconscious, open his airway and check to see if he is breathing normally.

1 Open airway

● Place one hand on the infant's forehead and gently tilt the head back.
● Lift the infant's chin using one finger of your other hand.
● Do not push on the soft part of the chin as it can block the airway.

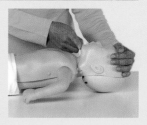

2 Look, listen, and feel for breathing

● Look along the chest for movement, listen for breathing, and feel for breath on your cheek for no more than 10 seconds.

If the infant is breathing normally,
● Check for life-threatening injuries.
● Hold him in the recovery position (opposite).

If the infant is not breathing,
● Begin rescue breathing (opposite).

Recovery position (infant)

If an unconscious infant is breathing normally, hold him so that his head lower than his body. This keeps his airway open and clear and his neck and spine aligned and stable.

1 Keep airway open

- Cradle the infant in your arms with his head lower than his body, to prevent him from choking on his tongue or inhaling his vomit.

✚ **CALL 911 OR LOCAL EMS**

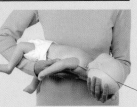

Head is lower than body

2 Monitor infant

- Monitor and record the infant's vital signs—level of response, pulse, and breathing (pp.20–1)— regularly until help arrives.

Rescue breathing (infant)

If an unconscious infant is not breathing normally, you will need to begin CPR—a combination of rescue breaths to get oxygen into the lungs and chest compressions.

1 Keep airway open

- Make sure the infant's head is tilted back and the chin is lifted.

2 Clear any obstructions

- Pick out any obvious obstructions from the mouth with your finger and thumb.
- Do not do a fingersweep of the mouth.

3 Give rescue breaths

- Take a normal breath and place your lips around infant's mouth and nose to form an airtight seal.
- Blow firmly and steadily for about one second; you should see the chest rise.
- Lift your mouth away from the infant's face and let the chest fall.
- Give two rescue breaths.

- If the chest does not rise and fall, check that his head is far enough back and that you have an effective seal around the infant's mouth and nose.

4 Begin chest compressions

- After two breaths (or attempts at breaths) begin chest compressions (p.52).

Pick out visible obstructions

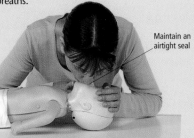

Maintain an airtight seal

INFANT LIFE-SAVING SEQUENCE

Check response

If infant does not respond,

Ask a helper to
✚ **CALL 911 OR LOCAL EMS**

Check breathing

If breathing, place in recovery position

OR

If not breathing normally,

Give two rescue breaths

Begin chest compressions and rescue breaths (CPR)

Repeat for two minutes and
✚ **CALL 911 OR LOCAL EMS**
if a call has not already been made

Continue CPR

Chest compressions (infant)

After two attempts at rescue breaths begin chest compressions (below) to circulate the blood with rescue breaths (p.52). If you are alone, do two minutes of CPR (five cycles) before you call the emergency services.

1 Give chest compressions

- Lay the infant on a firm, flat surface, either at roughly waist height or on the floor.
- Place the fingertips of your first two fingers on the center of his chest, just below the nipple line.
- Press down one-third to one-half of the depth of the infant's chest "push hard and fast." Release the pressure without removing your fingers from the breastbone. Let the chest come back up to its normal position.
- Press down on the chest 30 times in total at a rate of 100 times per minute.

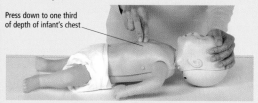

Press down to one third of depth of infant's chest

2 Repeat rescue breaths

- After you have given 30 chest compressions, tilt the infant's head, lift the chin, and give two more rescue breaths through the mouth and nose (p.51).

3 Alternate chest compressions with rescue breaths

- Continue the cycle of 30 compressions and two rescue breaths until emergency help arrives and takes over, the infant starts breathing normally, or you become so exhausted that you cannot carry on.

IMPORTANT
▶ If you are alone and the infant is not breathing, complete two minutes of CPR before taking the infant with you to call an ambulance.

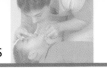

Choking adult

An object such as a piece of food stuck at the back of the throat can block the windpipe and result in choking. If the blockage remains, the victim may lose consciousness, so prompt first aid is vital. Follow the steps below for adults, and children over puberty; see page 54 for younger children, and page 55 for infants.

Your aims
▶ Clear obstruction from throat
▶ Get victim to the hospital if necessary

SIGNS AND SYMPTOMS
▶ With mild choking: red face and coughing
▶ With severe obstruction: cough is silent, victim is unable speak or breathe

1 Ask victim if he is choking

● If choking is mild and he is coughing, encourage him to continue.
● If the victim nods "yes," coughs silently, and stops beathing, the obstruction is severe and he needs help.

2 Prepare for abdominal thrusts

● Stand behind the victim and place a clenched fist with thumb side in over his upper abdomen just above the belly button.

3 Give abdominal thrusts

● Grasp your fist and pull inward and upward, up to five times.
● Check the mouth to see if the object has been dislodged. Remove the object or ask victim to spit it out.

Pull inward and upward

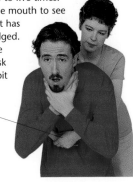

4 Repeat step 3

● If he is still choking after three sets of abdominal thrusts,

✚ **CALL 911 OR LOCAL EMS**

● Continue abdominal thrusts until medical help arrives, the victim spits the object out or he loses consciousness.

WARNING
▶ If the victim loses consciousness,
✚ **CALL 911 OR LOCAL EMS**

Open the airway, check breathing. Give chest compressions and rescue breaths (p.40–3) to try to dislodge the object.
▶ If given abdominal thrusts he must see a doctor.

Choking child

Young children can easily choke on food or small objects. Your priority is to remove the obstruction and clear the airway as quickly as possible. Follow the instructions below for children between the age of one and eight years.

Your aims
▶ Clear obstruction from throat
▶ Get child to the hospital if necessary

SIGNS AND SYMPTOMS
▶ With mild choking: red face, and coughing
▶ With severe obstruction: cough is silent, child is unable speak or breathe

1 Ask child if she is choking

● If choking is mild and she is coughing, encourage her to continue.
● If the child nods "yes," coughs silently, and stops beathing, the obstruction is severe and she needs help.
● Check the child's mouth and pick out any visible obstructions.

2 Prepare for abdominal thrusts

● Stand behind the child and place a clenched fist with thumb side in over her upper abdomen just below the ribs.

WARNING
▶ If the child loses consciousness
✚ **CALL 911 OR LOCAL EMS**
Open the airway, check breathing, and if not breathing, give chest compressions and rescue breaths (pp.46–9) to try to dislodge the object.

▶ If a child is given abdominal thrusts she must be seen by a doctor.

3 Give abdominal thrusts

● Grasp your fist with your other hand and pull inward and upward. Do this up to five times.
● Check the mouth and pick out any obstructions you can see.

Give five abdominal thrusts

Place first fist with thumb against abdomen

4 Repeat step 3

● If the child is still choking after three sets of abdominal thrusts,
✚ **CALL 911 OR LOCAL EMS**
● Continue abdominal thrusts until help arrives, the child spits the object out, or she loses consciousness.

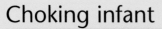

Choking infant

If an infant's airway is partially blocked, he may be distressed and coughing. If it is completely blocked, he will be unable to breathe or cough and will quickly become unconscious. For a choking infant (under 12 months), follow the instructions below.

> **Your aims**
> ▶ Clear obstruction from throat
> ▶ Get infant to the hospital if necessary

> **SIGNS AND SYMPTOMS**
> ▶ With mild choking: infant has red face, is able to cry and cough
> ▶ With severe obstruction: infant has difficulty crying, making any noise, and is unable to breathe

1 Give infant back blows

● If the infant is unable to cough or cry, sit down and lay him face down along your forearm.
● Give infant up to five sharp back blows with the heel of your hand.

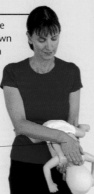

Give back blows with heel of your hand

3 Give chest thrusts

● Lay the infant face up on your arm, your lap, or on a firm surface.
● Give up to five downward thrusts to the chest.
● Check the mouth for any obstructions and pick them out.

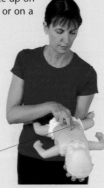

Use two fingers to give chest thrusts

2 Pick out any obstructions

● Check the infant's mouth.
● Remove any visible obstructions using your fingertips.

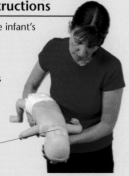

Look for obstructions in mouth

4 Repeat steps 1 to 3

● If the obstruction has still not cleared after three cycles of steps 1–3, keep the infant with you and
✚ **CALL 911 OR LOCAL EMS**
● Repeat steps 1–3 until help arrives, the child spits the object out, or she loses consciousness. .

> **WARNING**
> ▶ If the infant loses consciousness
> ✚ **CALL 911 OR LOCAL EMS**
> Open the airway, check breathing, and if not breathing, give chest compressions and rescue breaths (pp.50–2) to try to dislodge the object.

> **IMPORTANT**
> ▶ Do not put your fingers down the infant's throat to feel for, or attempt to remove, an obstruction.
> ▶ Do not use abdominal thrusts on an infant.

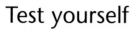
Test yourself

Now that you have read and studied the chapter on life-saving techniques, see if you can answer the questions below. After completing the questions, check your answers against the correct ones on page 144.

1 What does ABC stand for in the ABC of resuscitation?

A ....

B ....

C ....

2 Which organ pumps blood around the body?

....

....

3 What is the correct order for treating an unconscious victim?

Put him in recovery position ....

Open airway ....

Call ambulance ....

Check breathing ....

4 How long should it take to give a rescue breath?

One second ....

Two seconds ....

Three seconds ....

5 When and why is it good practice to use a face mask?

....

....

....

....

....

....

....

6 What does CPR stand for and what is it?

....

....

....

....

....

7 Which is the correct place to press down when giving chest compressions?

a Upper half of the chest .... ☐

b Lower half of the chest.................... ☐

c Center of the chest .... ☐

8 When starting CPR, how many chest compressions and rescue breaths should you give and in what order. At what rate should you give the chest compressions? Answer for an adult, child, and infant victim.

Adult ....

....

....

Child ....

....

....

Infant...

....

....

9 What is a defibrillator?

....

....

....

10 Which of the following indicate that a victim could be choking?

a Red face... ☐

b Swollen hands .... ☐

c Clutching the throat .... ☐

d Coughing .... ☐

e Rapid breathing through the mouth .... ☐

f Difficulty breathing....................... ☐

11 Which of the following techniques should not be used on a conscious infant who is choking?

Chest thrusts ....

Back blows ....

Abdominal thrusts ....

3 Wounds and bleeding

A wound is a break in the body's protective layer—the skin. This break allows germs to enter the body, causing possible infection and blood to escape. Severe blood loss is serious because oxygen is carried around the body by blood. If too much blood is lost, then insufficient oxygen is supplied to the tissues, resulting in a potentially life-threatening medical condition called shock.

Clear anatomical information explains what happens when blood vessels are damaged to help you understand why first-aid treatments are effective. This chapter clearly sets out general principles that apply to treating any wounds and bleeding. There are guidelines, too, for adapting the techniques when necessary for minor cuts and abrasions or serious wounds such as amputation.

Use the questionnaire on page 74 to test your understanding of the procedures described in this chapter.

Contents

Dealing with severe bleeding

Blood loss can be serious and should be controlled as soon as possible. If the victim loses a lot of blood, a condition called shock will develop, and eventually he will lose consciousness. If the bleeding is external, there will be a wound visible in the skin from which blood is escaping. Only approach the victim if it is safe to do so. Assess the wound, check for embedded objects, and ask the victim what has happened. Severe bleeding can be distressing, so explain what you are doing to reassure him. Make sure you avoid pressing on any foreign object in the wound.

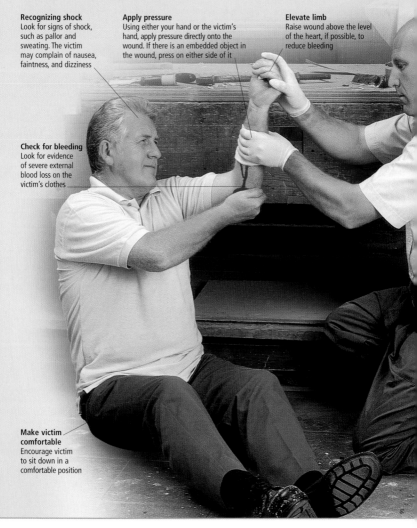

Recognizing shock
Look for signs of shock, such as pallor and sweating. The victim may complain of nausea, faintness, and dizziness

Apply pressure
Using either your hand or the victim's hand, apply pressure directly onto the wound. If there is an embedded object in the wound, press on either side of it

Elevate limb
Raise wound above the level of the heart, if possible, to reduce bleeding

Check for bleeding
Look for evidence of severe external blood loss on the victim's clothes

Make victim comfortable
Encourage victim to sit down in a comfortable position

Get a history
Ask the victim how the injury occurred

Check for danger
Make sure that the cause of injury does not pose any further threat and that there are no additional risks to you or the victim

What you should do

Your aims
▶ Control bleeding
▶ Prevent infection
▶ Prevent shock if possible
▶ Get victim to the hospital urgently

IMPORTANT
▶ Take care with hygiene—wear disposable gloves if available.
▶ Do not allow the victim to eat, drink, or smoke in case a general anesthetic is needed in the hospital.

1 Examine wound

● Check the wound to make sure there are no embedded objects (p.70).

2 Apply pressure to wound

● Press on the wound with your fingers or palm, ideally over a sterile dressing or clean pad. You can ask the victim to do this while you put on disposable gloves.
● If there is an embedded object, press on either side of the object.

3 Raise and support limb

● If the victim is bleeding from a limb, raise and support the limb above the level of his heart.

4 Dress wound

● Secure the dressing over the wound with a roller bandage.
● If blood seeps through, put on a second dressing.
● If blood seeps through the second dressing, remove both dressings and start again, making sure pressure is accurately applied over the wound.

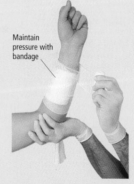

Maintain pressure with bandage

5 Check for shock

● Help the victim to lie down and watch for signs of shock (p.61).
● Call 911 or local EMS.
● Monitor and record the victim's vital signs—level of response, pulse, and breathing (pp.20–1)—regularly until help arrives.

Blood vessels and bleeding

In the body of the average adult, there are 10½ pints (6 liters) of blood, or about 1¾ pints (1 liter) of blood per 28lbs (13kg) of body weight, circulating around the body. The main component of blood is a fluid called plasma. This fluid contains red and white blood cells and also platelets, which help the blood to clot. Blood is carried around the body by vessels called arteries, capillaries, and veins. If blood vessels are damaged, they constrict at the site of the injury and the blood clotting process begins (below).

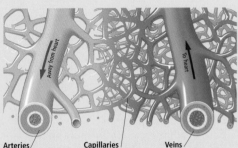

Arteries
These blood vessels have muscular walls through which blood travels at high pressure. Arteries carry blood containing oxygen from the heart to the tissues.

Capillaries
These tiny, thin-walled vessels connect arteries and veins. Their thin walls allow oxygen and nutrients to pass to the body tissues, and waste products such as carbon dioxide to be carried away.

Veins
Blood without oxygen is carried back to the heart through the veins, which have thinner, less muscular walls than the arteries.

How blood clots

A blood clot is the solidification of blood that occurs either spontaneously within a blood vessel or as the result of a leakage from the vessel. A clot that forms outside a blood vessel usually occurs in response to damage to that vessel. For example, at the site of a wound, blood leaks from the skin because the blood vessels beneath it are damaged and the blood then solidifies to form a clot (below). At the same time, the blood vessels constrict to limit the flow of blood to the wound.

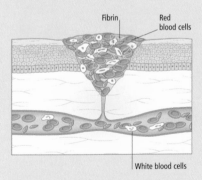

Fibrin   Red blood cells

White blood cells

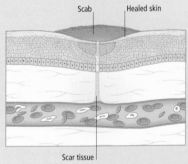

Scab   Healed skin

Scar tissue

Bleeding from a wound
Small blood cells called platelets clump together at the site of the wound. The platelets and damaged blood vessels then react to form a chemical called thrombin. This, in turn, reacts with a blood protein and creates fibrin filaments to form a mesh at the wound site.

Forming a protective scab
More platelets and red and white blood cells gather together inside the fibrin mesh. The fibrin filaments then contract and a clot is quickly formed. Eventually, the clot hardens and a protective scab forms over the site of the cut, which then heals and may leave a scar.

Shock

This life-threatening condition occurs when the circulation of blood around the body is reduced and vital organs, such as the brain and heart, do not get enough oxygen. Shock is most commonly caused by severe blood loss; it can also be the result of fluid loss due to burns, vomiting, or diarrhea, or the result of a severe allergic reaction (see Anaphylactic shock p.129). Emergency medical treatment is vital.

SIGNS AND SYMPTOMS
▶ Pale, cold, and clammy skin
▶ Nausea
▶ Rapid and then weak pulse
▶ Fast and shallow breathing
▶ Restlessness
▶ Yawning and sighing
▶ Thirst
▶ Gradual loss of consciousness; eventual death if treatment is not successful

Your aims	You will need
▶ Treat obvious causes of shock ▶ Improve circulation ▶ Get victim to the hospital urgently	▶ Blanket/coat ▶ Notepad and pen

1 Treat injuries

● Treat any obvious injuries, such as bleeding, burns, or broken bones.

2 Help victim lie down

● Help the victim to lie down.
● Raise his legs above the level of his heart if they are not injured.
● Reassure the victim.

3 Keep victim warm

● Protect the victim from extremes of temperature, if necessary by placing a blanket or coat around him.
✚ **CALL 911 OR LOCAL EMS**

4 Monitor victim

● Monitor and record the victim's vital signs—level of response, pulse, and breathing (pp.20–1)—regularly until help arrives.

Internal bleeding

● This can result from damage to an internal organ or from an injury that causes a major bone, such as the pelvis or a thighbone (femur), to break; both of these conditions can cause severe bleeding within the body.
● You should suspect internal bleeding if the victim is displaying signs of shock, if you notice a large amount of swelling around the site of the injury, or if the victim is experiencing a marked degree of tenderness around the abdomen.

IMPORTANT
▶ Do not allow the victim to eat or drink as he may later need a general anesthetic in the hospital.

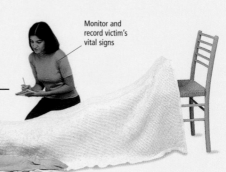

Monitor and record victim's vital signs

Cuts and abrasions

Small cuts and abrasions soon stop bleeding without treatment. However, any break in the skin, even a small one, can allow germs to enter the body. Germs are microorganisms, such as bacteria, that are carried by flies or by unwashed hands; if they are allowed to settle on an open wound, they can cause infection.

Your aims	You will need
▶ Stop wound from becoming infected ▶ Control any bleeding	▶ Disposable gloves ▶ Sterile gauze swabs or antiseptic wipes ▶ Adhesive bandage or sterile wound dressing ▶ Bandage

IMPORTANT
▶ Do not handle the open abrasion or cut with your fingers while you are treating the victim.
▶ Do not try to remove anything that is embedded in the wound; treat as described on p.70.
▶ Do not use cotton on or near an open wound because fibers may stick to the wound.

1 Rinse wound

● Help the victim to sit down.
● Put on disposable gloves, if available.
● Raise the injured part.
● Rinse the wound under cold running water to remove any dirt or grit.

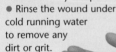

Rinse wound to remove any dirt

2 Clean around wound

● Using a fresh swab or wipe for each stroke, clean around the wound, working from the edge of the wound outwards.
● Carefully pick off any loose foreign matter, such as glass, metal, or gravel, from or around the wound.

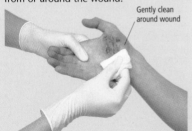

Gently clean around wound

3 Dry around wound

● Without disturbing the wound, gently dry the area around it with a gauze swab.

4 Cover wound

● For a small cut or abrasion, cover the injury with an adhesive bandage; make sure you do not touch the sterile part of the dressing.
● If the cut or abrasion is too large for an adhesive bandage, cover it with a sterile wound dressing and bandage.
● Advise the victim to rest the injured part and, if possible, to support it in a raised position.

Tetanus immunization

Tetanus is a serious infection caused by a bacterium that lives in the soil. Infection can be prevented by immunization. Always ask a victim with a cut or wound about his tetanus immunizations. Seek medical advice if:
● He has never had a tetanus injection.
● He does not know when he last had a tetanus immunization or how many injections he has had.
● It is more than 10 years since his last tetanus injection.

Bruising

This follows an injury and is caused by bleeding into the skin or into tissues beneath the skin. The area can become blue-black rapidly, or the bruise may take a few days to appear. Bruises that appear quickly will benefit from first aid. Elderly people and those taking blood-thinning (anticoagulant) drugs are likely to bruise particularly easily.

Your aim	You will need
▶ Reduce swelling	▶ Cold compress

1 Support injury

● Support the injured part in the most comfortable position for the victim.

2 Apply cold compress

● Place a cold compress (p.25) on the bruised area to reduce the blood flow to the injury and relieve pain.
● Press firmly on the compress and keep it in place for at least five minutes.

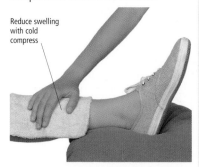

Reduce swelling with cold compress

WARNING
▶ A "black eye" is a bruise normally caused by a blow to the face. As it may also cause damage to the eye or skull, you should always seek medical advice.

Blisters

These result from friction or friction burns, which occur when the skin is rubbed repeatedly against a surface. Blisters develop when tissue fluid leaks from the damaged area and collects under the outer layer of the skin.

Your aims	You will need
▶ Relieve pain	▶ Soap and cold water
▶ Prevent infection	▶ Clean pad
	▶ Adhesive bandage or sterile wound dressing
	▶ Adhesive tape/ bandage

1 Clean affected area

● Wash the area carefully with soap and cold water and rinse with cold water.

2 Dry affected area

● Using a gentle patting action, dry the area and the surrounding skin very thoroughly with a clean pad.

3 Protect blister

● Carefully cover the blister with an adhesive bandage, or special blister dressing. Make sure the pad is larger than the blister.
● If the blister is very large, use a sterile wound dressing or a piece of nonfluffy material, secured with adhesive tape or a bandage.

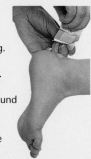

IMPORTANT
▶ Never deliberately burst a blister.

Crush injury

A crush injury is usually the result of a building site incident or a road accident. The injury may include a fracture as well as internal and external bleeding. If a victim is crushed for a prolonged length of time, body tissues—especially muscles—will be damaged, and when the pressure is released the victim will go into shock. Toxic chemicals will also build up in the crushed tissues and, if released suddenly into the circulation, they can cause kidney failure. Follow the instructions below if the victim has been trapped for less than 15 minutes; if the victim has been trapped for more than 15 minutes, follow the instructions given in the box at the bottom of the page.

Your aims	You will need
▶ Release victim	▶ Disposable gloves
▶ Treat any injuries	▶ Sterile wound
▶ Get victim to the	dressing/clean pad
hospital urgently	▶ Notepad and pen

1 Remove object

- Put on disposable gloves, if available.
- Remove the object, provided that it has not been there for more than 15 minutes.

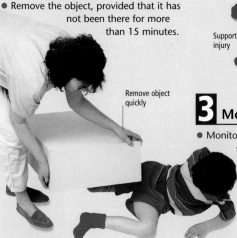

Remove object quickly

Support injury

2 Treat injuries

- Place a sterile wound dressing on any wounds and press firmly to control any bleeding (pp.58–9).
- Immobilize any fractures (pp.102–13).
- Treat the victim for shock (p.61).
- ✚ **CALL 911 OR LOCAL EMS**

3 Monitor victim

- Monitor and record the victim's vital signs—level of response, pulse, and breathing (pp.20–1)—regularly until help arrives.

If crushed for more than 15 minutes

IMPORTANT
▶ Do not release the victim if he has been crushed for more than 15 minutes.
✚ **CALL 911 OR LOCAL EMS**

- Act calmly and reassure the victim.
- Monitor and record the victim's vital signs—level of response, pulse, and breathing (pp.20–1)—regularly until help arrives.

Amputation

The complete or partial severing of a limb or digit (finger or toe) is known as amputation. The amputated part can, in many cases, be reattached by microsurgery, so it is important to get the victim and the severed part to the hospital as soon as possible. The victim is likely to suffer from shock (p.61) and will need to be treated.

Your aims	You will need
▶ Minimize blood loss	▶ Disposable gloves
▶ Treat for shock	▶ Sterile wound
▶ Get victim to the hospital urgently	dressing or pad and roller bandage
▶ Prevent deterioration of amputated part	▶ Notepad and pen
	For amputated part:
	▶ Kitchen film/ plastic bag
	▶ Soft fabric
	▶ Ice

1 Control bleeding

● Put on disposable gloves, if available.
● Raise the injured part, then place a sterile wound dressing or clean pad on the wound and press on it firmly to control the bleeding.
● If the digit or limb is partially severed, bring the parts together, wrap the dressing or pad around the wound, and then apply pressure over the wound.
● Make victim comfortable and treat for shock, if required (p.61).

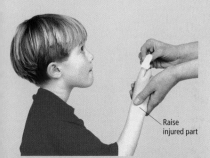

Raise injured part

WARNING
▶ Do not let the victim eat, drink, or smoke; he will need a general anesthetic for microsurgery.

2 Secure dressing

● Secure the dressing or pad with a roller bandage (p.26).
➕ **CALL 911 OR LOCAL EMS**

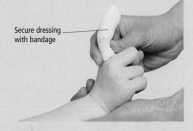

Secure dressing with bandage

IMPORTANT
▶ Tell the dispatcher that the victim has an amputation.
▶ If a digit has been amputated and the victim is not in shock, you could take him and the amputated part to the hospital yourself.

3 Monitor victim

● Monitor and record his vital signs— level of response, pulse, and breathing (pp.20–1)—regularly until help arrives.

Care of amputated part

● Do not wash the amputated part.
● Wrap the amputated part in plastic wrap or put it in a plastic bag.
● Wrap the package in soft fabric and place it in ice, but do not let it come into direct contact with the ice.
● Label the package with the victim's name and the time of injury.
● Give it to the emergency services.

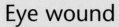

Eye wound

The eye can be injured by direct blows or by sharp splinters of grit or glass. Even a minor eye injury should be examined promptly by a doctor to prevent any loss of vision. It is important that the victim remains still during and after treatment.

Your aims	You will need
▶ Cover wounded eye	▶ Disposable gloves
▶ Get victim to the hospital urgently	▶ Gauze pad
	▶ Bandage

SIGNS AND SYMPTOMS
▶ Intense pain and fluttering of eyelid
▶ Obvious wound to, or bloodshot, eye
▶ Problems with vision
▶ Leakage of blood or clear fluid from eye

1 Keep victim still

● Help the victim to lie on his back, and cradle his head in your lap.
● Tell him not to move his eyes because this may cause further damage.
● Reassure the victim.

IMPORTANT
▶ Do not remove a foreign object in the eye (p.132).
▶ For chemical burns to the eye, see p.81.

2 Cover eye

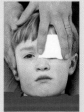

● Put on disposable gloves, if available.
● Cover the injured eye with a gauze pad.

✚ **CALL 911 OR LOCAL EMS**

● If medical help is delayed, secure the dressing in place with a bandage.

Scalp wound

The scalp, the skin covering the head, has many small blood vessels running close to its surface. For this reason, any wound to the scalp can result in profuse bleeding, making an injury appear more serious than it is.

Your aims	You will need
▶ Control bleeding	▶ Disposable gloves
▶ Get victim to the hospital	▶ Sterile wound dressings
	▶ Roller bandage

2 Help victim lie down

● Help the victim to lie down with her head and shoulders slightly raised.

✚ **TAKE OR SEND THE VICTIM TO THE HOSPITAL**

1 Control bleeding

● Put on disposable gloves, if available.
● Gently place a sterile wound dressing over the wound.
● Press firmly on the pad.
● Secure the dressing with a roller bandage.
● If blood shows through, secure another sterile dressing on top of the original one.

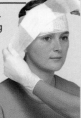

WARNING
▶ If the wound follows a blow to the head, treat as for head injury (p.93); monitor changes to level of consciousness.

✚ **CALL 911 OR LOCAL EMS**

▶ Monitor and record the victim's vital signs (pp.20–1) regularly until help arrives.

Nosebleed

Bleeding from the nose usually follows a blow to the nose, but it can occur without any apparent cause.

Your aims	You will need
▶ Control bleeding	▶ Tissues
▶ Prevent choking	

1 Ask victim to sit down

● Ask the victim to sit down and lean her head forward.
● Offer her tissues to wipe away blood.
● Loosen her collar if it is tight.

2 Pinch nose

● Tell her to pinch the soft part of her nose for 10 minutes and to breathe through her mouth.
● If the bleeding continues, pinch the nose again.
● While she is pinching her nose, tell her to spit out any blood in her mouth.
● Once bleeding stops, tell the victim not to blow her nose for several hours, as this may disturb the clot.

IMPORTANT
▶ If the nose is still bleeding after applying pressure for 30 minutes,

✚ **CALL 911 OR LOCAL EMS**

WARNING
▶ If yellowish, bloodstained fluid is coming from the nose and/or ear after a blow to the head, it could indicate a skull fracture.
▶ Gently help the victim to lie down as carefully as possible, and follow the first-aid action as described for head injury (p.93).

Ear wound

The usual cause of a bleeding ear is a burst eardrum, caused by a foreign object or a blow to the head.

Your aims	You will need
▶ Cover wound	▶ Disposable gloves
▶ Get victim to the hospital urgently	▶ Sterile wound dressing

IMPORTANT
▶ Do not attempt to plug the ear.
▶ Do not try to remove a foreign object.

1 Help victim lie down

● Help the victim to lie down with his head and shoulders raised.

2 Cover wound

● Put on disposable gloves, if available.
● Place a sterile wound dressing over the ear and lightly secure it with the bandage.

✚ **CALL 911 OR LOCAL EMS**

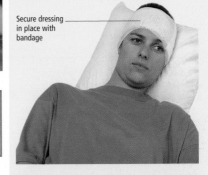

Secure dressing in place with bandage

✚ **CALL 911 OR LOCAL EMS**

▶ Monitor and record the victim's vital signs—level of response, pulse, and breathing (pp.20–1)—regularly until help arrives.

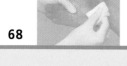

Mouth wound

Cuts to the tongue and lips are usually caused by the victim's own teeth. Bleeding from the mouth or a tooth socket may also occur straight after losing a tooth or some time after a tooth has been removed by a dentist.

Your aims	You will need
▶ Keep airway clear	▶ Disposable gloves
▶ Control bleeding	▶ Gauze pad

IMPORTANT
▶ Get medical or dental help if the mouth bleeds for longer than 30 minutes, and replace bloodsoaked gauze pads with fresh ones.
▶ Tell the victim not to drink anything hot for 12 hours after the bleeding has stopped.

1 Keep airway clear

● Help the victim to sit down.
● Lean her forward and toward the injured side to help the blood drain away and keep the airway clear.

2 Press on wound

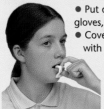

● Put on disposable gloves, if available.
● Cover the wound with a gauze pad.
● Ask the victim to press the pad onto the wound for 10 minutes.

If a tooth socket is bleeding

● Put a gauze pad over the socket. The pad should be thick enough to stop the top and bottom teeth meeting.
● Tell the victim to bite on this for 10 minutes.

Detail

Knocked-out tooth

If an adult tooth has been knocked out, it may be possible to be replant it, but this must be done by a dental practitioner.

Your aims	You will need
▶ Preserve tooth	▶ Disposable gloves
▶ Get victim to dentist	▶ Gauze pad
	▶ Milk or water

1 Preserve tooth

● Put on disposable gloves, if available.
● Handle the tooth by its crown (not the root) and place it in a container with some milk or water if there is no milk.
● Place a gauze pad in the tooth socket to help stop bleeding and ask the victim to press on the pad.
● Never try to replant a tooth.

2 Get victim to dentist

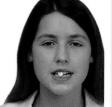

● Take or send the victim to a dental practitioner.

Apply pressure to control bleeding from socket

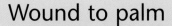

Wound to palm

It can be difficult to apply pressure to the wound to control the bleeding when it is in the palm of the hand. If there is nothing embedded in the wound, treat the injury as shown below. If an object is embedded, treat as described on pages 70–1.

Your aims	You will need
▶ Control the bleeding	▶ Disposable gloves
▶ Get victim to the hospital	▶ Sterile wound dressing
	▶ Triangular bandage

1 Apply pressure

- Put on disposable gloves, if available.
- Check the wound to make sure that nothing is embedded in it.
- Apply direct pressure to the wound; either you or the victim can do this.
- Raise the hand above the level of the heart.

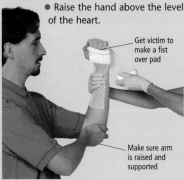

Get victim to make a fist over pad

Make sure arm is raised and supported

2 Cover wound

- Put a sterile dressing on the wound. Ask the victim to clench his fist over the pad.
- Roll the bandage around the clenched fist to secure the dressing, leaving the thumb exposed. Tie a square knot (p.22) over the fingers.

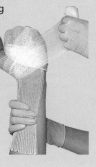

3 Check circulation

- Check the circulation in the thumb on the injured arm (see Roller bandages p.26).
- If the circulation is restricted, loosen the bandage and check the circulation again.

4 Secure arm in sling

- Support the victim's arm in an elevation sling (p.29).
- Recheck the circulation in the victim's thumb.

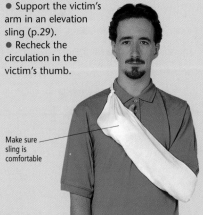

Make sure sling is comfortable

5 Get victim to a hospital

✚ **TAKE OR SEND THE VICTIM TO THE HOSPITAL**

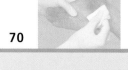

Embedded object

If an object is embedded or stuck in a wound, never try to remove it. This is because the object may be plugging the wound, preventing bleeding, and also you may do more damage by pulling it out. Instead, protect the area with gauze and place a dressing spare rolled-up bandages around the object, then hold them in place with another bandage. This will maintain enough pressure to control the bleeding without pressing directly on to the wound or the object.

Your aims	You will need
▶ Control bleeding	▶ Disposable gloves
▶ Protect wound from infection	▶ Piece of gauze
▶ Immobilize affected area	▶ Bandages for padding and to cover wound
▶ Get victim to the hospital	

WARNING
▶ If the object is large or embedded near a vital organ or an eye,

✚ **CALL 911 OR LOCAL EMS**

1 Control bleeding

● Put on disposable gloves, if available.
● Help the victim to lie down.
● Pinch the edges of the wound together around the embedded object to control severe bleeding.
● If possible, raise and support the injured part of the body.

2 Cover wound

● Drape a piece of gauze gently over the wound and the protruding object to reduce the risk of infection.

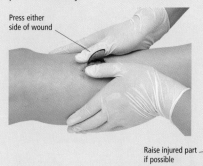

Press either
side of wound

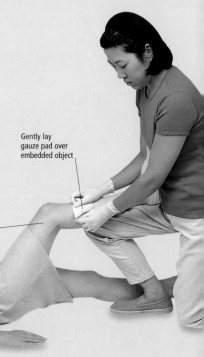

Gently lay
gauze pad over
embedded object

Raise injured part
if possible

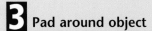

3 Pad around object

- Very carefully, place padding either side of the protruding object to protect the wound and control the bleeding.
- Build up enough padding so that you can bandage over the embedded object without pressing down on it.
- Make sure that you do not pull down on the embedded object as you position the padding.

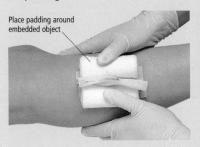

Place padding around embedded object

4 Bandage above and below object

- Place one end of a bandage over the part of the padding nearest to you.
- Make two straight turns with the bandage around the victim's limb.
- Pass the bandage under the limb and wrap it around the other side of the padding.

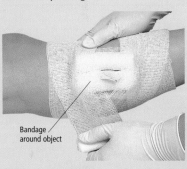

Bandage around object

If the object does not protrude

- Place the padding either side of the object and wrap the bandage directly over the padding but without pressing down on the object.

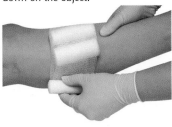

5 Secure dressing

- Continue the diagonal turns around the injury on either side of the padding until the dressing is firm. Secure the bandage.
- Keep the injured part raised, where possible, and keep it as still as you can.

✚ TAKE OR SEND VICTIM TO THE HOSPITAL

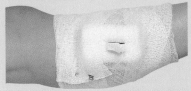

IMPORTANT

▶ Find out about the victim's tetanus immunizations. Seek medical advice if the victim has never had a tetanus injection, does not know when he was last injected or how many injections he has had, or it is more than 10 years since his last tetanus injection (p.62).

Splinters

Any tiny pieces, or splinters, of wood, glass, or metal are rarely clean. If they become embedded in the skin they may cause infection. If a splinter is sticking out of the skin, remove it with tweezers, as shown below. If the end of the splinter is not visible, seek medical help because it is easy to push a splinter even further into the skin.

Your aims	You will need
▶ Remove splinter from skin	▶ Disposable gloves
	▶ Cold water
▶ Prevent wound from becoming infected	▶ Tweezers
	▶ Match or lighter

SIGNS AND SYMPTOMS
- ▶ Pain where splinter went into skin
- ▶ Cause of injury may be close by
- ▶ Splinter visible in skin

1 Clean wound

- Put on disposable gloves, if available.
- Rinse the area around the splinter with cold water.
- Make sure that you do not touch the wound with your fingers.

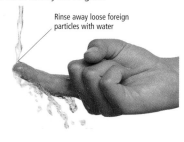

Rinse away loose foreign particles with water

2 Sterilize tweezers

- Sterilize the tweezers by passing them through the flame of a match or lighter.
- Allow the tweezers to cool.
- Do not wipe the soot off or touch the end of the tweezers.

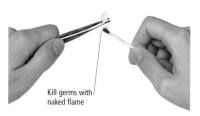

Kill germs with naked flame

3 Pull out splinter

- Grasp the splinter with the tweezers as close to the skin as possible.
- Carefully draw out the splinter, making sure that you pull it out at the same angle that it went into the skin.

Pull out splinter in straight line

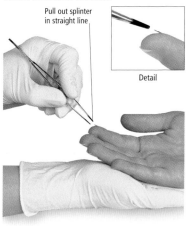

Detail

IMPORTANT
- ▶ Never dig into the skin to get at a splinter.
- ▶ If the splinter breaks, do not continue trying to remove it.
- ▶ Find out about the victim's tetanus immunizations (p.62).

Fishhook injury

When a fishhook is embedded in the skin, do not try to remove it unless there is no medical help available. Simply bandage around the hook before making sure that the victim receives medical help. Embedded fishhooks carry a risk of infection.

Your aims	You will need
▶ Get medical help	▶ Disposable gloves
▶ Prevent further injury by padding around embedded fishhook	▶ Scissors
	▶ Gauze pads
	▶ Bandage
	▶ Adhesive tape
If medical help is not available:	If medical help is not available:
▶ Remove hook	▶ Wirecutters
	▶ Sterile wound dressing

1 Help victim sit down

● Help the victim to sit in a comfortable position and reassure him.

2 Cut fishing line

● Put on disposable gloves, if available.
● Cut the fishing line as close as possible to the hook.

3 Build up pads of gauze

● Carefully put pads of gauze around the embedded fishhook.
● Build up pads of gauze until you can bandage over the hook without pushing it further into the skin (pp.70–1).

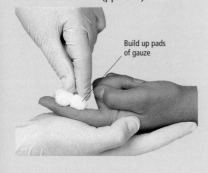
Build up pads of gauze

4 Bandage over gauze padding

● Bandage over the hook and padding, taking care not to press down on the hook.
● Secure the bandage with adhesive tape.

➕ **TAKE OR SEND VICTIM TO THE HOSPITAL**

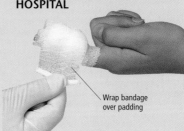
Wrap bandage over padding

If medical help is not available

Try to remove a fishhook only if medical help is not available.
● If the barb of the hook is not visible, push it further into the skin until it pokes through.
● Cut off the barb with wirecutters.
● Never try to remove a fishhook if you cannot cut off the barb as you will damage the underlying tissues.
● Withdraw the hook by its eye (the end that attaches to the fishing line).
● Clean the wound, and apply a sterile wound dressing and bandage.
● Find out about the victim's tetanus immunizations (p.62).

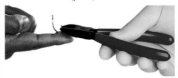

Test yourself

Now that you have read and studied the chapter on first-aid treatments for wounds and bleeding, see if you can answer the questions below. Check your answers against the correct ones on page 144.

1 Which three steps in the following list should you take to control bleeding?
 a Raise the wound above the level of the heart............................ ☐
 b Give chest thrusts............................ ☐
 c Apply pressure to the wound .... ☐
 d Cool the victim with a wet sponge....................................... ☐
 e Apply a dressing and bandage to the wound.................................. ☐

2 What should you do if blood seeps through a dressing?
....
....

3 What are the three types of blood vessels that carry blood around the body?
1...
2...
3...

4 Which medical condition will develop if a large amount of blood is lost?
....
....

5 What should you do to prevent an abrasion becoming infected?
....
....
....
....
....

6 The first aider in the picture is monitoring a victim with shock. What three things should she be checking?
1...
2...
3...

7 Why should you put a cold compress on a bruise?
....
....

8 What two actions should you tell a victim with a nosebleed to do to stop the bleeding?
1...
2...

9 What should you do if a victim loses one of his adult teeth?
 a Replant the tooth and get the victim to see a dental practitioner ....☐
 b Keep the tooth in milk get the victim to a dental practitioner ....☐
 c Throw the tooth away ....☐

10 If a yellowish, bloodstained fluid comes from the victim's nose or ear, what might it indicate?
....

11 How do you control bleeding if there is an embedded object in a wound?
....
....
....

4 Environmental injuries

This chapter focuses on treating injuries and illnesses caused by environmental factors, such as extremes of heat and cold. Fire, electricity, hot liquids, and chemicals can all burn the skin, which protects the body and helps to maintain a normal body temperature. Extremes of temperature can also affect the skin and other body functions, especially in young children and elderly people.

This section of the book explains how to treat different types of burn and sets out the priorities for dealing with localized injuries, such as sunburn and frostbite, and generalized conditions, such as dehydration and heatstroke.

Use the questionnaire on page 88 to test your understanding of first aid for environmental injuries.

Contents

Dealing with severe burns

A burn or scald damages the skin and can lead to infection. Severe burns also cause loss of fluids, which will lead to shock (p.61). Scalds are burns caused by extremes of moist heat, such as boiling water or steam. When dealing with a burn, you need to act quickly to reduce the effect of the heat on the skin and prevent germs getting into the burned area and causing infection. A severe burn requires urgent hospital treatment to minimize any subsequent damage (see When a victim needs medical help, p.78).

WARNING

▶ Any burning injury that is accompanied by smoke may lead to smoke inhalation and irritation of the airways and lungs, which may cause breathing difficulties.

▶ If the victim is having breathing difficulties,

✚ **CALL 911 OR LOCAL EMS**

Be ready to begin resuscitation if necessary (pp.36–52).

Watch for shock
Look out for any signs of shock, such as pallor and sweating; the degree of shock will depend on the depth and extent of the burn

Get a history
Ask the victim what caused the burn or scald

Cool burn
Flood burn with water

Blistered skin
If there are blisters, do not attempt to burst them because they provide a barrier to infection

Severe pain
The victim will complain of pain if the surface of the skin is affected but deep burns are not usually painful because the nerve endings are destroyed

Swelling around injury
This will develop very quickly around any burn

Redness around injury
The skin will become red very quickly after an injury from a burn

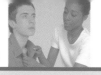

Check for danger
Approach the victim only if it is safe to do so. Check that whatever caused the incident represents no further danger to either of you

Give reassurance
Explain to the victim what you are doing to help reassure her and keep her calm

What you should do

Your aims
▶ Cool burn
▶ Prevent infection
▶ Treat any shock
▶ Get medical help

IMPORTANT
▶ Do not apply creams, sprays, ointments, or adhesive tape.
▶ Do not touch the burned area.
▶ Do not overcool as this may lead to hypothermia.
▶ Do not remove any clothing sticking to the burn.

1 Cool burn

● Flood the burn with copious amounts of cold water until the burning sensation eases.

2 Cover burn

● Put on disposable gloves, if available.
● Remove any burned clothing unless it is sticking to the burn.
● Remove restrictions such as rings, bracelets, or belts before swelling starts.
● Cover the burned area with a sterile wound dressing, clean cloth, plastic bag, or plastic wrap to prevent infection.

3 Treat shock

● Watch for signs of shock developing and treat accordingly (p.61).
● Help the victim to lie down.
● Constantly reassure the victim.

4 Get medical help

● Seek urgent medical advice for all severe burns.
● Call 911 or local EMS if necessary, or advise the victim to see a doctor.
● Monitor the victim's vital signs—level of response, pulse, and breathing (pp.20–1)—regularly until help arrives.

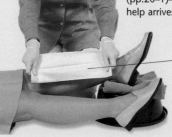

Make sure dressing is large enough to cover entire wound

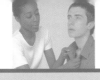

Types of burn

The severity of a burn depends on the type of burn and on the size of the area of skin that is affected. There are three types of burn: first- , second-, and third-degree burns (below). A victim with a third-degree burn may not feel any pain because the nerve is damaged, which may make you and the victim think that the burn is not as serious as it really is. Burns can cause fluid loss and lead to shock (p.61); the more extensive the burn, the greater the risk of shock developing. See the box below for detailed guidelines of when to get medical help for a burn. However, if you are in any doubt about the seriousness of a burn, always seek medical advice.

How burns affect the skin

The skin is made up of two layers: the outermost visible layer called the epidermis and the inner dermis underneath. Skin has many functions, one of which is to protect the body from invasion by germs. A burn or scald can break this protective barrier, allowing germs to enter the body and lead to infection.

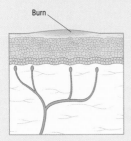

Burn

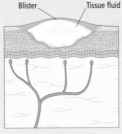

Blister   Tissue fluid

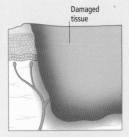

Damaged tissue

First-degree burn
This type of burn affects only the epidermis, causing redness and swelling. It is not serious unless it covers a large area (below). With prompt first aid, a first-degree burn should heal in a few days.

Second-degree burn
This deeper burn destroys the epidermis. The skin turns red and is covered with blisters. This type of burn is painful but usually heals well. If, however, it covers a large area, it can be serious, even fatal.

Third-degree burn
This type of burn destroys the epidermis and damages the dermis. It affects nerves, tissues, muscles, and blood vessels. The skin appears pale or charred. Third-degree burns require urgent medical attention.

When a victim needs medical help

Any infant or child with a burn should have urgent hospital treatment, regardless of the size of the burn. For adults, always seek medical help for any of the following:
- Third-degree, or full-thickness, burns.
- Burns on the face, hands, feet, or genital area.
- Burns that reach right around an arm or a leg.
- Second-degree burns that cover an area about the size of the palm of the victim's hand.
- First-degree burns that cover an area equivalent to the size of five of the victim's palms.
- Burns of mixed depth.

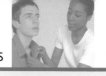

Minor burns and scalds

The majority of small burns and scalds are the result of incidents in the kitchen. A burn may be caused by touching a hot oven or iron, while a scald may be the result of spilling boiling water on the skin or coming into contact with steam from a kettle.

Your aims	You will need
▶ Cool burn	▶ Cold water
▶ Relieve pain and swelling	▶ Disposable gloves
▶ Prevent burn becoming infected	▶ Sterile wound dressing

SIGNS AND SYMPTOMS
▶ Reddening of skin
▶ Pain in area of burn
▶ Blister, smaller than victim's palm

IMPORTANT
▶ If you are at all concerned about the severity of the burn, make sure the victim gets medical help.

1 Cool burn

● Flood the area of the burn with copious quantities of cold water for at least 10 minutes or until the burning feeling stops.
● If water is not available, use any cold liquid, such as canned drinks.

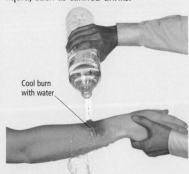

Cool burn with water

3 Cover burn

● Cover the burn with a sterile wound dressing or a clean, nonfluffy pad (p.24) to minimize the risk of infection. Alternatively cover the burn with a clean plastic bag, clean tea towel, clean sheet, or plastic wrap. Discard the first piece of film to make sure the wrap you use to cover the burn is as clean as possible.
● Tie the bandage loosely over the dressing to hold it in place.

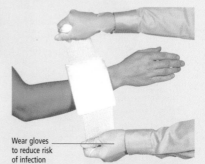

Wear gloves to reduce risk of infection

2 Raise limb

● Put on disposable gloves, if available.
● Raise the limb to reduce swelling.
● Remove any constricting jewellery or clothing before the area starts to swell.

WARNING
▶ Do not put any lotions, creams, ointments, or sprays on the burn as they might introduce infection.
▶ Do not put on any dressing that will stick to the burned area because it will be difficult to remove without causing further damage.

▶ Do not burst any blisters or touch the burned area. A small blister does not usually need any treatment, but if it bursts, apply a nonadhesive sterile wound dressing that extends beyond the edges of the blister. Leave the dressing in place until the blister heals.

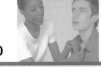

Face and head burns

Burns to the face, and in the mouth or throat, are particularly serious because they can cause the victim's airway to become swollen very quickly, making breathing difficult. If the burns are in the mouth or throat, you can usually see external signs of burning, such as soot around the mouth. For all these burns, emergency medical help is vital.

Your aims	You will need
▶ Get victim to the hospital urgently	▶ Cold water
▶ Keep airway open	▶ Towel
▶ Treat for shock if necessary	▶ Disposable gloves
	▶ Sterile wound dressing

SIGNS AND SYMPTOMS
▶ Very painful mouth, throat, and head
▶ Difficulty breathing
▶ Damaged skin and/or soot around mouth
▶ Shock may develop

1 Call 911 or local EMS

● Call the emergency services immediately.
● Tell the dispatcher that you suspect burns to the airway and that the victim is having difficulty breathing.

WARNING
▶ If the victim is unconscious, open the airway and check breathing. Put him in the recovery position if he is breathing. Be ready to begin resuscitation if necessary (pp.36–52).

2 Improve air supply

● Do anything you can to improve the victim's air supply, such as loosening tight clothing around the neck.
● Treat for shock, if necessary (p.61).

Burns to the head

● Keep the burned area cool; if possible, use a bottle or watering can or something similar to pour water gently over the head. Put a towel around the victim's shoulders to catch the water.
● If the burn is near the throat, nose, or mouth, be ready to begin resuscitation (pp.36–52).
● Put on disposable gloves, if available, and place a dressing on the burn, but do not bandage it in place; if necessary, hold the dressing on until help arrives.

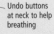

Undo buttons at neck to help breathing

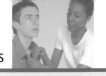

Chemical burns

Many chemicals used in the home or in the workplace can cause serious damage to the skin. Always act quickly to wash the chemical off and protect yourself as you treat the victim. Make sure any contaminated water can drain away freely.

Your aims	You will need
▶ Wash chemical away	▶ Disposable gloves
▶ Get victim to the hospital	▶ Cold water
	▶ Sterile wound dressing

SIGNS AND SYMPTOMS
▶ Chemicals near victim
▶ Stinging pain
▶ Discoloration, swelling, and blistering of skin
▶ Shock may develop

1 Wash chemical off skin

● Put on disposable gloves, if available.
● Hold the injured part under cold running water for at least 20 minutes to wash away the chemical.
● Take any contaminated clothing off the victim while you are flooding the affected area with water.

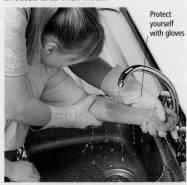

Protect yourself with gloves

2 Cover wound

● After washing the area, cover the burn with a sterile wound dressing.
● If necessary, treat the victim for shock (p.61).

✚ **TAKE OR SEND VICTIM TO THE HOSPITAL**

Burns to the eye

If the victim has been splashed in the eye with a chemical, his eye will water and the surrounding area will become swollen. He may also not be able to open his eye. Act quickly to wash the chemical out of the victim's eye.
● Put on disposable gloves, if available.
● Positioning the head so that contaminated water does not run down the face, hold the affected eye under gently running cool water for at least 20 minutes.
● If the victim is still in pain, continue pouring water over the eye.
● Take or send the victim to a hospital.
● Once the pain has eased, ask the victim to hold a sterile wound dressing lightly over the eye.

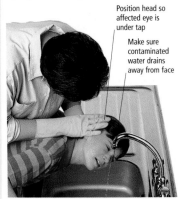

Position head so affected eye is under tap

Make sure contaminated water drains away from face

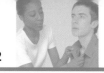
Electrical burns

These burns can occur when an electrical current passes through the body and may be visible at the point where electricity enters or leaves the body. Electrical burns at home are caused by low-voltage current, so it is safe to switch the current off; do not approach a person who has suffered high-voltage burns (p.11).

Your aims	You will need
▶ Treat visible burns and any shock ▶ Get victim to the hospital urgently	▶ Cold water ▶ Sterile wound dressing or clean, nonfluffy material ▶ Scissors

SIGNS AND SYMPTOMS
▶ Casualty may be unconscious
▶ Swollen, charred skin at site of contact
▶ Shock may develop
▶ High-voltage burn may leave brownish residue on skin

1 Turn off electricity

● Where possible, turn off the electricity at the main switch or fuse box to break the contact between the victim and the electrical supply. Alternatively, pull out the plug from the socket.

2 Cool burn

● Pour cold water over the burn for at least 10 minutes or until the burning feeling stops.
● Carefully cut away any clothing from around the burn.

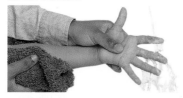

WARNING
▶ Do not touch the victim if you cannot break the contact between him and the electrical supply as you may be electrocuted. Follow the advice on p.11.
▶ An electrical burn may lead to unconsciousness. If the victim is unconscious,

✚ **CALL 911 OR LOCAL EMS**

Open the airway and check breathing. Put him in the recovery position if he is breathing. Be ready to begin resuscitation if necessary (pp.36–52).

3 Cover burn

● Place a sterile wound dressing carefully over the burn.
● If you do not have a wound dressing, place some clean, nonfluffy material such as a clean folded triangular bandage or plastic wrap over the affected area. Or put a clean plastic bag over a burned hand or foot, securing the bag with tape.

✚ **CALL 911 OR LOCAL EMS**

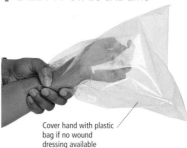

Cover hand with plastic bag if no wound dressing available

4 Reassure victim

● Reassure the victim and, if necessary, treat for shock (p.61).

IMPORTANT
▶ If the victim has suffered a high-voltage burn (p.11), do not approach him until the current has been officially switched off. Keep yourself and bystanders at a safe distance of 60 ft (18m) from the source of electricity.

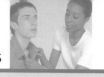

Sunburn

Overexposure to the sun's rays will result in sunburn. At high altitudes, it is possible to get sunburned even if the sky is overcast; reflected off snow, the effects of sunlight are intensified and particularly damaging. Using a sunlamp may also cause sunburn. If a victim has severe sunburn he may also suffer from heatstroke (p.85).

Your aims	You will need
▶ Take victim out of sun ▶ Relieve discomfort and pain	▶ Cold water and towel/sponge ▶ Drinking water ▶ Calamine lotion/aftersun cream

SIGNS AND SYMPTOMS
▶ Red and very hot skin
▶ First-degree burns
▶ Blistering
▶ Heatstroke

IMPORTANT
Prevention is better than cure:
▶ Wear sunscreen when in the sun.
▶ Do not stay in the sun for too long.
▶ Limit exposure to the sun by wearing a hat, and uncover only small areas of the body at a time.

1 Take victim into shade

● Cover the victim's skin with light clothing or a towel and move him out of the sun and into the shade.

2 Cool burn

● Remove the clothing.
● Cool the burned area by gently dabbing on cold water with a towel or sponge.

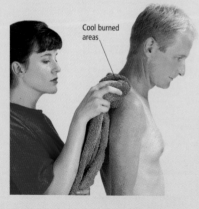

Cool burned areas

3 Give water

● Give the victim frequent sips of water.

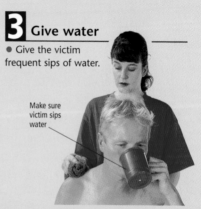

Make sure victim sips water

4 Apply soothing lotion

● If the sunburn is mild, apply calamine or aftersun cream to the skin.

WARNING
▶ If the skin is blistered or the sunburn covers a large area,

✚ **TAKE OR SEND VICTIM TO THE HOSPITAL**

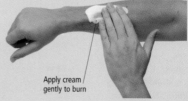

Apply cream gently to burn

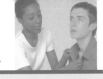
Dehydration

Water makes up 50–60 percent of the body of a healthy adult. Normally, there is a balance between the amount of water the body takes in and the amount the body excretes. Dehydration occurs when the body has too little water. It is common in babies who are ill, elderly people, and those suffering from diarrhea, vomiting, or a fever. Exercise, particularly if it is strenuous or takes place in hot weather, can result in dehydration.

Your aims	You will need
▶ Replace lost water	▶ Drinking water,
▶ Treat cause	preferably nonfizzy
▶ Get medical help if necessary	▶ Notepad and pen

SIGNS AND SYMPTOMS
▶ Feeling thirsty
▶ Nausea
▶ Muscle cramps

1 Give sips of water

● Give the victim frequent small sips of water to replace lost body fluids. Continue until he stops feeling thirsty. If possible, use only still water, not fizzy.

2 Find cause of dehydration

● Look for any other illness, such as fever or vomiting and diarrhea, to try to discover why the victim is dehydrated.
● Prevent any strenuous exercise until the victim has recovered.

3 Monitor victim

● Monitor and record the victim's vital signs—level of response, pulse, and breathing (pp.20–1)—regularly.
● If the victim does not recover or his condition worsens, get medical help.

Heat exhaustion

This condition is caused by an abnormal loss of salt and water from the body through excessive sweating. It usually develops gradually and is more likely to affect people who are not accustomed to hot and humid conditions and those who are already ill.

Your aims	You will need
▶ Cool victim down	▶ Drinking water or nonfizzy drink
▶ Replace lost fluid	
▶ Get victim to the hospital urgently	

SIGNS AND SYMPTOMS
▶ Cramp-like pains and/or headache
▶ Pale, moist skin
▶ Fast, weak pulse
▶ Slightly raised temperature

1 Help victim lie down

● Help the victim to lie down in a cool place.
● Raise his legs to improve blood flow.

2 Give water

● Give the victim plenty of water to drink or a nonfizzy drink to replace lost fluids.
✚ CALL 911 OR LOCAL EMS

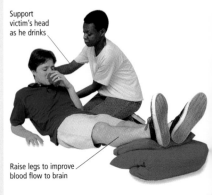

Support victim's head as he drinks

Raise legs to improve blood flow to brain

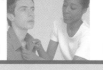

Heatstroke

This potentially dangerous condition occurs when the body is unable to cool itself by sweating, due to illness or prolonged exposure to heat and humidity. The use of drugs such as ecstasy can raise the body temperature and may lead to heatstroke. Common in very hot climates, the condition can also occur during hot spells in milder climates. People who exercise in hot weather are particularly prone to heatstroke.

Your aims	You will need
▶ Lower victim's body temperature as quickly as possible	▶ Cushions/pillows
	▶ Two large sheets
▶ Get victim to the hospital urgently	▶ Water and spray
	▶ Fan (preferably electric but keep it away from the water)
	▶ Thermometer
	▶ Notepad and pen

SIGNS AND SYMPTOMS
- ▶ Restlessness
- ▶ Headache
- ▶ Dizzy feeling
- ▶ Flushed and very hot skin
- ▶ Rapid loss of consciousness
- ▶ Fast, strong pulse
- ▶ Raised body temperature, which may reach 104°F (40°C) or higher

1 Get victim to cool place

- Help the victim to lie down in a cool place and remove his outer clothes.
- Place cushions or pillows behind his head to make him more comfortable.

2 Cool with water and fan

- If available, wrap the victim in a cold, wet sheet and keep it wet, or sponge his body down with cold or tepid water.

✚CALL 911 OR LOCAL EMS
- Fan the victim until his temperature falls to 100.4°F (38°C) under the tongue, or 99.5°F (37.5°C) under the armpit (p.21).

3 Change sheet

- When the victim's temperature has fallen to a safe level, replace the wet sheet with a dry one.

4 Monitor victim

- Monitor and record his vital signs—level of response, pulse, and breathing (pp.20–1)—regularly until help arrives.

Make victim comfortable with cushions or pillows

Spray sheet continually with water to keep it wet

Wrap victim in wet sheet

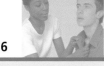

Hypothermia

When the body temperature drops below 35°C (95°F), hypothermia sets in. It is often caused by wearing unsuitable clothes in cold weather or by being in cold water for too long. It can also result from being in a poorly heated or unheated room. Elderly people are especially at risk because they are less aware of changes in temperature. Infants, too, are susceptible to hypothermia because they are not capable of regulating their own body temperatures. Active rewarming should only be started if you are a long way from medical help and there is no risk of further cold.

Your aims	You will need
▶ Prevent victim's body temperature falling any further	▶ Warm, dry clothes
	▶ Blankets, survival bag, or sleeping bag
▶ Make victim warmer	▶ Insulating material, such as bracken
▶ Get medical help if necessary	▶ Warm drink

SIGNS AND SYMPTOMS
▶ Loss of consciousness
▶ Very cold, pale skin
▶ Shivering
▶ Clumsiness, irritability
▶ Slurred speech
▶ Slow breathing, weak pulse, and lethargy

1 If far from medical help rewarm victim

● Advise the victim to stop any physical activity immediately and rest.
● If a long way from medical help (and there is no risk of further cold), replace wet clothing with warm, dry clothes.
● If possible, send someone to get help; don't leave the victim.

2 Shelter victim

● If possible, make a shelter to protect the victim from the weather.
● Wrap her in a survival bag, sleeping bag, or blanket.
● Lay her down on dry, insulating material, such as dry heather or bracken.

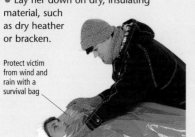

Protect victim from wind and rain with a survival bag

3 Give victim warm drink

● If possible, give the victim a warm drink, such as warm milk or hot chocolate. Do not give her alcohol.
● Reassure and comfort her.

Give victim a warm drink

4 Check for frostbite

● If the victim appears to have frostbite (opposite), treat her accordingly.

5 Call 911 or local EMS

● Arrange to get the victim to the hospital on a stretcher. Do not let her walk.

WARNING
▶ If the victim is unconscious, open the airway and check breathing. Put her in the recovery position if she is breathing. Be ready to begin resuscitation if necessary (pp.36–52).

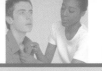

For a victim indoors

✚ GET MEDICAL HELP

● If you are a long way from a medical facility, and there is no risk of further cold, start rewarming the victim.

● If a victim has been brought inside wearing wet clothes, replace these with warm, dry clothes as soon as possible.

● If the victim is young and fit and can climb into a bath on her own, rewarm her in the bath, making sure the water temperature is not too hot—about 104°F (40°C).

● If the victim is elderly or an infant, wrap her in blankets to rewarm her.

● Put the warmed victim into bed and make sure she is well covered. Cover her head for additional warmth.

● Do not use a hot-water bottle or an electric blanket to warm a victim.

● Give victim warm drinks, soup, or high-energy foods, such as chocolate. Do not give any alcohol to drink.

● Stay with the victim until her skin becomes warm and returns to its normal color.

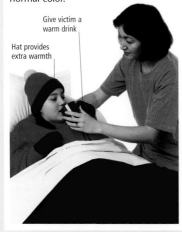

Give victim a warm drink

Hat provides extra warmth

Frostbite

Intense cold causes frostbite, resulting in parts of the body, such as the fingers or toes, becoming frozen. It may be accompanied by hypothermia (opposite).

SIGNS AND SYMPTOMS
▶ Prickling pain, followed by gradual loss of feeling
▶ Skin feels hard and turns white, then blue, and finally black

Your aims	You will need
▶ Get victim to the hospital	▶ Gauze bandage
▶ Warm affected area slowly if help not easily	

1 If far from medical help warm affected area

● If you are in a shelter, gently remove any tight or constrictive clothing, such as gloves or boots, and rings, from affected part.

● Get the victim to put his hands in his armpits or put his feet in your armpits.

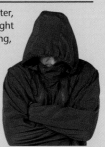

2 Cover affected area

● Cover the frostbitten part with a gauze bandage to protect it and keep it covered until color and feeling return to the skin.

✚ TAKE OR SEND VICTIM TO THE HOSPITAL

IMPORTANT
▶ Always warm the affected part slowly—never use a source of heat such as a hot-water bottle.
▶ Do not thaw a frostbitten foot if the victim needs to walk any further.
▶ Do not try to rewarm the area if there is a chance of refreezing, or you are near a medical facility.

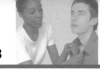

Test yourself

Now that you have read and studied the chapter on first-aid treatments for environmental injuries, see if you can answer the questions below. Check your answers against the correct ones on page 144.

1 What are your aims when treating a burn?
....
....
....

2 Name the three types of burn.
1..
2..
3..

3 What is the greatest risk from extensive burns?
....
....

4 When treating a burn, what should you not do?
....
....
....
....

5 Suggest some household items that can be used to cover a burn if you do not have a sterile wound dressing or pad.
....
....
....

6 What external signs might indicate burns to the mouth or throat?
....
....
....

7 How long should you cool a burn caused by heat and what is the risk to the victim of cooling it for too long?
....
....
....

8 How long should a chemical burn to the skin be held under cold running water?
....
....

9 What should your first action be when treating an electrical burn?
....
....

10 An athlete is feeling unwell after running a half-marathon on a hot summer's day. What might be the problem?
....
....

11 Name at least five signs or symptoms that indicate that a victim has hypothermia.
1..
2..
3..
4..
5..

12 What are your aims when treating a victim with frostbite?
....
....
....

5 Disorders affecting consciousness

This chapter describes first aid for injuries or conditions that affect consciousness. It begins by outlining the first-aid priorities for dealing with someone who has collapsed, explaining why it is important to carefully monitor a victim who is not fully conscious.

Easy-to-follow anatomical information helps you understand the effects that impaired consciousness can have on the body. This is followed by first-aid guidelines for the injuries or conditions that can lead to loss of consciousness: head injury, stroke (in which there is bleeding or a blood clot in the brain), fainting (which happens when insufficient oxygen-rich blood reaches the brain), and seizures (in which there is an electrical imbalance in the brain).

Use the questionnaire on page 100 to test your understanding of first aid for disorders affecting consciousness.

Contents

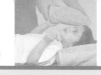
Dealing with a collapsed person

Some injuries and illnesses can result in a victim becoming dazed, confused, or even unconscious. The victim may be wide awake and alert, completely unresponsive to outside stimulation, or somewhere between these two extremes. If you are dealing with a victim who is not fully conscious, monitor any change in her level of response (p.20), especially any deterioration, because she could become unconscious at any time.

IMPORTANT
▶ If you suspect the victim has a neck or spinal injury, try to leave her in the position in which you found her. If you need to place her in the recovery position (p.38 adults; p.47 children), keep her head and neck in alignment with the body.

Get a history
If the victim is alert enough, ask what happened. If the victim is not alert, ask any bystanders what happened and listen carefully to what they say

Speak to the victim
Does she respond to simple questions or is she confused and unable to speak clearly?

Look for external clues
Check for clues such as a special bracelet or necklace, worn by people with conditions that may affect the level of consciousness, for example epileptic seizures or diabetes mellitus

Check breathing
Note whether the victim's breathing is noisy, difficult, or apparently normal

Look at her eyes
Assess how alert the victim is by checking if her eyes are open and moving

Check for danger
Look out for any hazards before you help the victim. Approach her only when you are sure that you are not in any danger

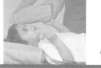

WARNING
▶ If the victim becomes unconscious,

✚ CALL 911 OR LOCAL EMS

Open the airway and check breathing. Be ready to begin resuscitation if necessary (pp.36–52).

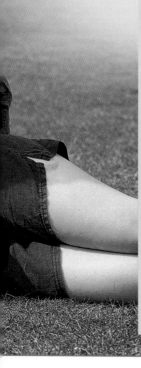

Find cause of injury
Visually examine the victim from head to toe. Look for an obvious cause of injury or a preexisting condition. For example, check whether she has fallen against something that may have caused a head injury

What you should do

Your aims
▶ Assess victim's level of consciousness and monitor any change
▶ Look for possible causes
▶ Arrange removal to the hospital if necessary

IMPORTANT
▶ Do not leave victim unless you have to go for help.
▶ Do not move victim unnecessarily.
▶ Do not allow victim to eat, drink, or smoke.
▶ Do not shake an infant or child to check consciousness.

1 Check response

● Assess the victim's level of response by following the AVPU code (p.20).
● If the victim loses consciousness, call 911 or local EMS. Open the airway, check breathing. Be ready to begin resuscitation (pp.36–52).
● If the victim is conscious, ask her what happened or if she has any known injury or illness.

2 Check her breathing

● Note the rate, depth, and quality of the victim's breathing (p.21).
● Listen especially for breathing difficulties.

3 Help victim sit or lie down

● Help the victim to sit or lie down in a comfortable position. If she is very dazed, help her to lie down rather than sit her in a chair because she may fall off a chair.

4 Do head-to-toe survey

● Examine the victim from head to toe for any injuries or illnesses (pp.18–19) and treat them accordingly.
● Look for warning signs, such as a special bracelet or necklace indicating a preexisting condition.
● Call 911 or your local EMS if necessary.

5 Monitor victim

● Monitor and record the victim's vital signs—level of response, pulse, and breathing (pp.20–1)—regularly until help arrives.

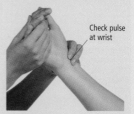

Check pulse at wrist

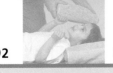

The nervous system

This is the system that controls body functions, such as consciousness, breathing, and movement, as well as detecting and responding to information coming from outside and inside the body. The nervous system consists of the brain and spinal cord (central nervous system) and a network of nerves branching from this system (peripheral nervous system). Any injury or illness that affects the nervous system is potentially serious because it may affect a victim's level of consciousness.

How the nervous system works

The brain contains millions of interconnected nerve cells, which control thought, sensation, movement, and functions such as breathing. The main function of the spinal cord is to convey high-speed electrical signals between the brain and the "wire-like" peripheral nerves.

The peripheral system has three divisions: sensory nerves that send information to the brain and spinal cord from sensory cells, for example in the eyes, ears, and skin; motor nerves that carry signals from the brain that allow us to move our muscles voluntarily; and autonomic nerves, which control involuntary, or "automatic," body functions, such as breathing, heartbeat, and digestion.

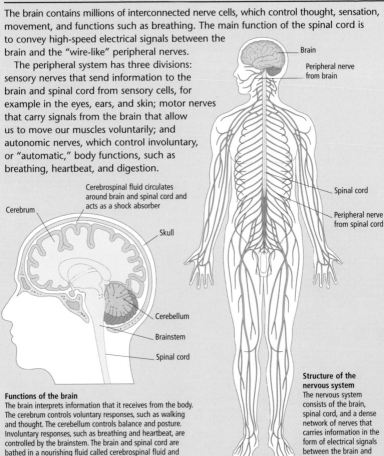

Functions of the brain
The brain interprets information that it receives from the body. The cerebrum controls voluntary responses, such as walking and thought. The cerebellum controls balance and posture. Involuntary responses, such as breathing and heartbeat, are controlled by the brainstem. The brain and spinal cord are bathed in a nourishing fluid called cerebrospinal fluid and surrounded by protective membranes called meninges.

Structure of the nervous system
The nervous system consists of the brain, spinal cord, and a dense network of nerves that carries information in the form of electrical signals between the brain and the rest of the body.

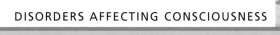

Head injury

Any blow to the head can cause a fracture of the skull and/or concussion or bleeding inside the skull leading to compression of the brain. If the victim shows any of the signs and symptoms that are listed below or on pages 94 and 95, the injury may be life-threatening. Call the emergency services. Treat a conscious victim as described below. For an unconscious victim, see the box below.

Your aims	You will need
▶ Assess victim carefully	▶ Notepad and pen
▶ Get medical help	

SIGNS AND SYMPTOMS
▶ Period of unconsciousness
▶ Yellowish, bloodstained fluid from ear or nose
▶ Bruising around eyelid or white part of eye
▶ Bleeding scalp
▶ Exposed skull
▶ Enlarged or different-sized pupils
▶ Unusually slow pulse rate

1 Check responses

● Check the victim's level of response using the AVPU code (p.20).
● If the victim is conscious and responsive, help her to sit or lie in a comfortable position. Continue to monitor her level of response.

IMPORTANT
▶ Always suspect a spinal injury (p.110) with anyone who has had a head injury.

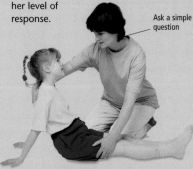

Ask a simple question

2 Get medical help

● Advise the victim to seek medical help if she later develops a headache, blurred vision, nausea, or excessive sleepiness.
● If the victim does not recover fully or if, after an initial recovery, her level of response deteriorates,
✚ **CALL 911 OR LOCAL EMS**
● If there is a yellowish, bloodstained fluid coming from the nose or ear, suspect a skull facture and
✚ **CALL 911 OR LOCAL EMS**

For an unconscious victim

● Ask a bystander to
✚ **CALL 911 OR LOCAL EMS**.
● If possible, leave the victim in the position in which you found her.
● Open the victim's airway using the jaw-thrust method (see For an unconscious victim p.111) in case she has a spinal injury, and check her breathing. Be ready to begin resuscitation if necessary (pp.36–52).

● If the victim is breathing and you need to leave her to call for help, put her in the adapted recovery position (box p.39).
● Monitor and record her vital signs— level of response, pulse, and breathing (pp.20–1)—regularly until help arrives.
● If she makes a rapid recovery, check her responses every 10 minutes and watch for signs of deterioration.

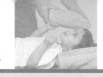

Concussion

This is usually caused by a blow to the head, which "shakes" the brain inside the skull, but it can also result from indirect force, such as landing heavily on your feet. The victim will be dazed and confused but probably for only a few minutes. Concussion is always followed by a complete recovery. If the victim later complains of symptoms such as a headache or blurred vision, advise her to seek medical help.

Your aims	You will need
▶ Make sure victim recovers fully ▶ Get victim looked after by responsible person ▶ Get medical help	▶ Notepad and pen

SIGNS AND SYMPTOMS
▶ Blow to head
▶ Short period of being dazed and confused
▶ Dizziness
▶ Nausea
▶ Brief loss of memory
▶ Headache

1 Help victim sit or lie down

● Help the victim to sit or lie down in a comfortable position.

IMPORTANT
▶ Always suspect a spinal injury (p.110) with anyone who has had a head injury.

2 Check responses

● Check the victim's level of response using the AVPU code (p.20).
● Monitor and record her vital signs—level of response, pulse, and breathing (pp.20–1)—regularly. Pay particular attention to her level of response.
● Treat any associated injuries.

3 Stay with victim

● When the victim has recovered, make sure someone responsible stays with her for the next few hours.
● If the injury has occurred during a sporting activity, do not allow her to continue playing the sport without first getting medical advice.

4 Get medical help

● Advise the victim to seek medical help if she later suffers from a persistent headache, nausea and vomiting, blurred vision, or excessive sleepiness.

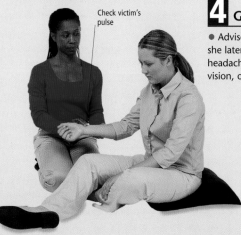

Check victim's pulse

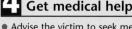

WARNING
▶ If the victim does not recover completely after a short time, if her level of response deteriorates after an initial recovery, or if there is an accompanying neck or other serious injury,

✚ **CALL 911 OR LOCAL EMS**

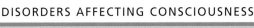
Compression

A heavy blow to the head can cause bleeding inside the skull or swelling of the injured part of the brain. This disturbs the brain's normal activity, resulting in a very serious, life-threatening condition called cerebral compression. The victim will probably need urgent medical treatment or even surgery. Treat a conscious victim as described below. For an unconscious victim, see the box at the bottom of the page.

Your aims	You will need
▶ Get victim to the hospital urgently ▶ Reassure victim ▶ Monitor victim	▶ Notepad and pen

1 Call 911 or local EMS

● Call the emergency services immediately.

2 Help victim sit or lie down

● Help the conscious victim to sit or lie down in a comfortable position and reassure her.

3 Monitor victim

● Monitor and record the victim's vital signs—level of response, pulse, and breathing (pp.20–1)—regularly until medical help arrives.

SIGNS AND SYMPTOMS

▶ Deteriorating level of response
▶ History of head injury
▶ Severe headache
▶ Unequal pupil size
▶ Weakness and/or paralysis down one side of body or face
▶ Change in behavior
▶ Noisy breathing
▶ Slow, strong pulse
▶ High temperature and flushed face

WARNING

▶ Compression may develop immediately after a head injury, a few hours later, or even days later.
▶ Compression can also be caused by a stroke (p.96), brain tumor, or infection.

IMPORTANT

▶ Always suspect a spinal injury (p.110) with anyone who has had a head injury.
▶ Do not let the victim eat, drink, or smoke—she may need a general anesthetic later in the hospital.

For an unconscious victim

● Ask a bystander to
➕ **CALL 911 OR LOCAL EMS**.
● If possible, leave the victim in the position in which you found her.
● Open her airway using the jaw-thrust method (see For an unconscious victim p.111), and check her breathing. Be ready to begin resuscitation if necessary (pp.36–52).
● If the victim is breathing and you need to leave her to call an ambulance, put her in the recovery position (p.38 adults; p.47 children; p.51 infants).

● Monitor and record her vital signs—level of response, pulse, and breathing (pp.20–1)—regularly until help arrives.

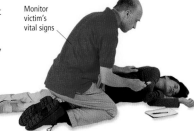

Monitor victim's vital signs

Stroke

A stroke occurs when the flow of blood in the brain is disrupted by a clot or bleeding from a damaged blood vessel. Strokes can be minor, in which case a full recovery is possible, or they can be major and possibly fatal. The severity of the stroke depends on the extent of the damage and where in the brain it has occurred. If you suspect a person has suffered a stroke, call the emergency services immediately. Treat a conscious victim as described below. For an unconscious victim, see the box at the bottom of the page.

Your aims	You will need
▶ Keep victim comfortable	▶ Damp flannel
▶ Get victim to the hospital urgently	▶ Notepad and pen

SIGNS AND SYMPTOMS
- ▶ Severe, sudden headache
- ▶ Dizziness and confusion
- ▶ Gradual or sudden loss of consciousness
- ▶ Paralysis down one side of body, with weak limbs and drooping of one side of face

1 Support head and shoulders

- Help the victim to lie down.
- Make sure her head and shoulders are slightly raised.

IMPORTANT
▶ Do not allow the victim to have anything to eat or drink because she may choke.

2 Tilt victim's head

- Tilt the victim's head towards the weaker side to allow fluid to drain out.
- Wipe her face with a damp flannel if she dribbles.

✚ CALL 911 OR LOCAL EMS

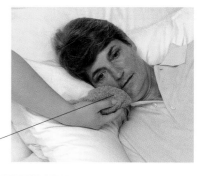

Wipe away saliva with damp flannel

For an unconscious victim

- Ask a bystander to
✚ CALL 911 OR LOCAL EMS.
- Open the victim's airway and check breathing. Put her in the recovery position if she is breathing, making sure her airway stays open. Be ready

to begin resuscitation (pp.36–52).
- Monitor and record her vital signs—level of response, pulse, and breathing (pp.20–1)—regularly until help arrives.

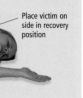

Place victim on side in recovery position

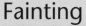
Fainting

A person faints when the amount of blood flowing to the brain is temporarily reduced, leading to a brief loss of consciousness. This can be caused by excessive pain but it can be the result of extreme emotion or standing still for a long time in a hot atmosphere—moving the feet and/or changing position can prevent this. If you give the correct first aid, the victim will usually recover quickly and completely.

Your aims
▶ Make sure blood reaches brain
▶ Make victim comfortable
▶ Reassure victim after recovery

SIGNS AND SYMPTOMS
▶ Feeling weak, faint, giddy, and possibly nauseous
▶ Very pale skin
▶ Slow pulse
▶ Loss of consciousness

WARNING
▶ If the victim does not recover quickly, put her in the recovery position (p.38 adults; p.47 children; p.51 infants) and

✚ **CALL 911 OR LOCAL EMS**

1 Raise legs above heart

● Help the victim to lie down.
● If she has already fainted, open her airway and check her breathing (p.37).
● Raise her legs above heart (chest) level.

Raise legs above heart level

Loosen tight clothing

2 Get fresh air to victim

● Loosen tight clothing around the neck, chest, and waist.
● Open any windows and ask bystanders not to crowd the victim.

3 Reassure victim

● Once the victim starts to recover, reassure her constantly and help her to sit up slowly.
● Treat any associated injuries.

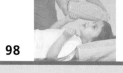
Seizures in adults

The most likely cause of a person suffering from a seizure is epilepsy, which is the result of electrical activity in the brain being disturbed. Epileptic seizures may be sudden and dramatic (below) or quite minor, with the victim looking as if she is daydreaming. Many people prone to epileptic seizures carry a warning card or wear a MedicAlert bracelet.

Your aims	You will need
▶ Protect victim from injury	▶ Soft padding, such as towel/pillow
▶ Reassure victim when she recovers	

SIGNS AND SYMPTOMS
▶ Sudden loss of consciousness
▶ Rigid body
▶ Convulsive jerking movements
▶ Relaxation of muscles at end of attack

1 Clear space around victim

● If possible, try to ease the victim's fall.
● Clear a space around her so that she does not hurt herself, and protect her from any danger.
● Keep calm and let the seizure run its course; there is nothing you can do to stop it.

2 Protect head

● If possible, place padding, such as towels or pillows, under or around her head to prevent injury (do this very carefully as it is easy to frighten someone who is having a seizure).
● Carefully loosen any tight clothing.

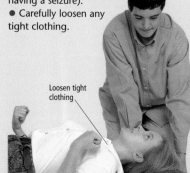

Loosen tight clothing

Place padding under head

3 Place in recovery position

● When the jerking stops, open the airway and check the breathing.
● Put her in the recovery position (p.38 adults; p.47 children; p.51 infants).

4 Reassure victim

● After the attack, remain with the victim until she has fully recovered. Monitor and record her vital signs (pp.20–1) regularly.

WARNING
▶ If the seizure lasts more than five minutes, if unconsciousness lasts more than 10 minutes, if the victim has repeated seizures and/or she does not regain consciousness, or if this is her first seizure,
✚ **CALL 911 OR LOCAL EMS**

IMPORTANT
▶ Do not try to hold the victim down or stop the seizure.
▶ Do not put anything in the mouth.
▶ Do not give the victim anything to eat or drink during a seizure.

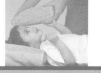

Seizures in young children

Young children tend to suffer from seizures when they are between the ages of one and four. They are generally caused by a high temperature (fever), serious tummy upset, fright, or temper. Although seizures can look very alarming, they are not usually dangerous, and problems rarely occur afterwards.

Your aims	**You will need**
▶ Protect child from injury ▶ Prevent temperature from rising further ▶ Get child to the hospital urgently	▶ Soft padding, such as towel/pillow ▶ Notepad and pen

SIGNS AND SYMPTOMS
▶ Flushed and sweating face
▶ Very hot forehead
▶ Stiffening and arching of back
▶ Eyes rolled upward
▶ Child may hold breath, resulting in bluish tinge to face
▶ Brief loss of consciousness

1 Protect child

● Place padding such as towels or pillows around the child to prevent her from injuring herself by a sudden movement.

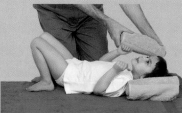

2 Cool child

● Remove the child's clothing and any bedclothes to prevent her temperature from rising further.
● Make sure there is a good supply of cool fresh air around her.

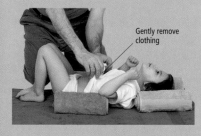

Gently remove clothing

3 Cover with sheet

● When the seizure stops, help the child to lie on her side if possible. Cover her with a sheet.
● Reassure her.
✚ **CALL 911 OR LOCAL EMS**
● Monitor and record the child's vital signs (pp.20–1)—regularly until help arrives.

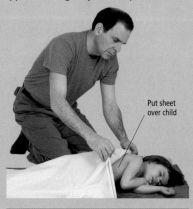

Put sheet over child

IMPORTANT
▶ Take care not to overcool the child.
▶ If the child loses consciousness,
✚ **CALL 911 OR LOCAL EMS**
Open airway and check breathing (p.46). If she is breathing put her in the recovery position (p.47).

Test yourself

Now that you have read and studied the chapter on first-aid treatments for disorders affecting consciousness, see if you can answer the questions below. Check your answers against the correct ones on page 144.

1 Why are injuries that affect the brain a cause for concern?
....
....

2 What five conditions might any head injury be accompanied by?
1..
2..
3..
4..
5..

3 How would you recognize compression?
....
....

4 How would you recognize concussion?
....
....

5 What should you do if a victim becomes unconscious?
....
....
....

6 Which of the following can cause a stroke?
a A blood clot in an artery in the heart .... ☐
b A blood clot in an artery in the brain .... ☐
c Bleeding from a damaged blood vessel in the brain .... ☐
d A blood clot in the lungs .... ☐

7 What is fainting?
....
....
....

8 Which of the following should you do when an adult victim is having an epileptic seizure?
a Make sure the victim's mouth is kept open.................. ☐
b Try to give the victim a sip of cool water .... ☐
c Clear a space around the victim so that he does not hurt himself....... ☐
d Send the victim back to work as soon as the seizure is over........... ☐
e Try to hold the victim tightly........... ☐

9 What are the tahree most important actions to take when a child is having a seizure?
1..
2..
3..

10 If you are waiting for medical help to arrive, what three things should you monitor regularly until it arrives?
1..
2..
3..

6 Bone, joint, and muscle injuries

This chapter describes first aid for injuries that affect the bones, joints, and the muscles that move them. The section begins by outlining your priorities for dealing with a suspected broken bone, because it can be very difficult for a first aider to differentiate between the different types of injury and this is the safest course of action.

There are easy-to-follow descriptions of the potential injuries: broken bones, sprained joints, dislocated joints, and strained muscles. This is followed by first-aid procedures for injuries to different parts of the body, from a broken jaw and cheekbone to rib, leg, and ankle injuries. Head injuries such as skull fractures are not dealt with in this chapter; they are covered in the section dealing with disorders affecting consciousness (see Head injury p.93).

Use the questionnaire on page 114 to test your understanding of first aid for bone, joint, and muscle injuries.

Contents

Dealing with a broken bone

Bones are normally very strong, but they can break or crack if they are struck or twisted (p.104). Injuries can also occur if bones at a joint are pulled out of their normal position, if the ligaments that support the joints are torn, or if the muscles are torn (p.105). It can be difficult to distinguish between a bone, joint, or muscle injury without an X-ray or a scan, so if you are in any doubt, treat the injury as a broken bone. You need to protect the victim from further injury or damage by keeping him as still as possible until help arrives.

WARNING
▶ Do not move the victim unnecessarily.
▶ If it is necessary to move the victim, enlist the help of others and plan the move before you start. Make sure the injured part is secured and supported.

Check for danger
Make sure there are no further risks to you or the victim. Remove the ladder if it is safe to do so

Get a history
Ask the victim what has happened. He may tell you he heard or felt a bone break

Keep victim still
Tell the victim to stay still and make sure he understands how important it is not to move

Watch for shock
Look for signs of shock, such as pallor and sweating. The victim may complain of feelings of nausea, faintness, and dizziness

Pain and tenderness
The victim may tell you that he is in great pain and that the area around the injury is tender

Swelling around injury
The affected area may appear swollen and bruised; however, this may not be evident at first

Check for deformity
The affected part of the body may appear deformed compared to the other side of the body

Give reassurance
Explain to the victim what you are doing to help reassure him and keep him calm

What you should do

Your aims
▶ Prevent further injury
▶ Get victim to hospital
▶ Treat any shock

IMPORTANT
▶ If the victim is unconscious and you suspect a neck injury, use the jaw-thrust method to open the airway (p.111).

1 Support injured limb

● Leave the victim in the position found.
● Secure and support the injured part by hand or by using rolled-up blankets or bandages depending on the site of injury.
● If the victim has fallen from a height, suspect that he has a spinal injury so support his head and neck at all times to prevent further injury.
● Cover any wound with a sterile wound dressing or clean pad.
● Check the circulation in a limb after applying any bandages (see Roller bandages p.26).

2 Get victim to a hospital

● The site and extent of the injury will determine how the victim should be transported to the hospital: for example, if it is an arm injury, you may be able to take him by car.
● If you suspect injury to the spine or neck, always call 911 or your local EMS.

3 Treat shock

● Look for signs of shock and treat the victim accordingly (p.61).

4 Monitor victim

● Monitor and record the victim's vital signs—level of response, pulse, and breathing (pp.20–1) —regularly until help arrives.
● Reassure him and tell him what is happening.

Support head and neck to prevent movement

IMPORTANT
▶ Do not allow the victim to eat, drink, or smoke as a general anesthetic may be needed at the hospital.

Types of bone, joint, and muscle injury

Injuries to the bones, joints, and muscles include fractures, dislocated joints, sprains, and strains. A fracture is a broken or cracked bone. A joint becomes dislocated when one of its bones is pulled out of its normal position. A sprain happens when the ligaments (the fibrous bands that hold bones together at a joint) become torn. A strain is an overstretched muscle or tendon (the fibrous band that attaches muscle to bone).

> **IMPORTANT**
> ▶ It can be difficult to tell the difference between bone, joint, and muscle injuries. Finding out how the incident happened (p.17) may indicate the type of injury to suspect. If in doubt, it is safest to treat the injury as a broken bone and seek medical help.
> ▶ Do not move the injured part of the victim unnecessarily as you may cause further damage to blood vessels, tissues, or internal organs.
> ▶ Do not give the victim anything to eat or drink as he may need a general anesthetic later.

Broken bones

A considerable force is needed to break a bone unless the bone is already weakened by disease. The force can be direct, indirect, or twisting. A direct force, such as a kick, will break the bone at the point of impact. An indirect force will cause a break some distance from the point of impact; for example, a fall onto an outstretched hand may break the collarbone. A twisting force can also break a bone; this can occur when a foot that is stuck twists in a way that breaks the ankle.

Broken bones are very painful. If a large bone breaks, there will be internal bleeding from broken blood vessels in the bone. If a protective bone, such as a rib, is broken, there is a risk of damage to internal organs. Children—because their bones are still growing and flexible—may have greenstick fractures, in which a bone cracks, splits, or bends.

The injury can be stable, in which the broken ends stay in place, or unstable, in which the ends are likely to move and may break through the skin. If the ends do break through the skin, or there is a wound, the break is open. If the skin is intact, the break is closed.

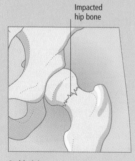
Impacted
hip bone

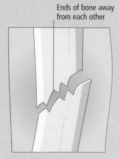
Ends of bone away
from each other

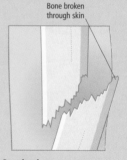
Bone broken
through skin

Stable injury
In a stable injury, either the bone is not completely broken, or the broken ends are impacted (wedged into each other), and the risk of further immediate damage or bleeding is small.

Unstable injury
If the broken ends of the bone can slide past each other, it is an unstable injury. Damage to the surrounding tissues and organs is possible, especially if the injured part is moved.

Open break
In an open break, the skin is broken, sometimes with the bone protruding. Bleeding is likely, and there is a risk of infection. If the skin is intact, the injury is known as a closed break.

Joint injuries

The main injuries that can affect joints are sprains and dislocations, both of which are very painful and can be slow to heal. A sprained joint generally happens when a sudden or unexpected wrenching movement stretches or tears a ligament that supports a joint. This type of injury is especially common around the ankle and may happen when a victim twists his ankle after misjudging a step.

A dislocated joint can result from a strong force that wrenches one of the bones of a joint out of the normal position. This type of injury is most common at the shoulder, jaw, and joints in the finger or thumb—a dislocated thumb is a particularly common skiing injury. A dislocated joint in the backbone can be very serious because there may be damage to the spinal cord (p.92). In some instances, a dislocation of the shoulder or hip may damage nerves in the region of the affected joint.

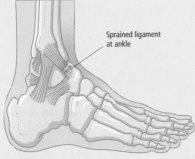

Sprained ligament
at ankle

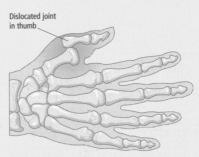

Dislocated joint
in thumb

Sprained joint
When a joint is sprained, there is often swelling and bruising around the joint. The injury may also cause the joint to have a limited range of movement.

Dislocated joint
In this type of injury, the joint will appear to be misshapen, or deformed, when compared to other similar joints. There may also be swelling and bruising around the affected joint.

Muscle injuries

The muscles that move the skeleton are attached to bones by tendons. A muscle or tendon can be pulled or "strained." This type of injury often occurs at or near to the point where the muscle and tendon join to each other. A strained muscle may have just a few or many fibers torn. A strained tendon may be torn completely. These injuries are also painful.

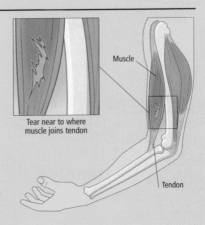

Muscle

Tear near to where
muscle joins tendon

Tendon

Torn muscle and tendon
This type of injury has extensive, deep bruising, leading to severe pain and discomfort. A torn muscle or tendon usually takes a long time to heal.

Jaw injury

A broken jaw is usually caused by a direct blow to the jaw. Rarely, a blow to one side of the jaw can also fracture the other side.

SIGNS AND SYMPTOMS
▶ Pain when speaking, chewing, or swallowing
▶ Bloodstained saliva
▶ Displaced teeth
▶ Swelling and/or unevenness along jaw

Your aims	You will need
▶ Keep airway open	▶ Soft pad
▶ Get victim to the hospital	

1 Keep airway open

● Lean the victim forward to let any fluid drain away from his mouth.
● Ask the victim to spit out any loose teeth or dentures. Keep them to give to the emergency service personnel (p.68).

2 Support jaw

● Ask the victim to hold a soft pad loosely against his jaw.

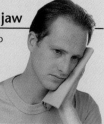

3 Get victim to a hospital

✚ **TAKE OR SEND VICTIM TO THE HOSPITAL**

WARNING
▶ If the victim is seriously injured or is not fully conscious, put him in the recovery position (p.38 adults; p.47 children) with the injured side down and a soft pad under his head.

✚ **CALL 911 OR LOCAL EMS**

Cheek and nose injury

A blow of considerable force to the face, such as occurs in a road accident, is commonly the cause of a fractured cheekbone or nose.

SIGNS AND SYMPTOMS
▶ Swelling and bruising
▶ Pain around affected area

Your aims	You will need
▶ Reduce swelling	▶ Cold compress
▶ Get victim to the hospital	

1 Apply cold compress

● Place a cold compress (p.25) on the injured area to reduce the swelling.

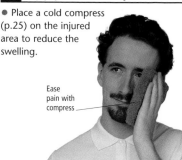

Ease pain with compress

2 Treat nosebleed

● If necessary, treat the victim for a nosebleed (p.67).

3 Get victim to a hospital

✚ **TAKE OR SEND VICTIM TO THE HOSPITAL**

IMPORTANT
▶ If there is a yellowish, bloodstained fluid leaking from the nose, assume the victim has a skull fracture and treat accordingly (p.93).

Collarbone injury

A broken collarbone is usually the result of indirect force, for example from falling onto an outstretched hand. This transmits force along the victim's forearm and upper arm to the collarbone. It can also be caused by a direct blow. Collarbone injuries often occur in young people as a result of sporting activities.

Your aims	You will need
▶ Immobilize collarbone	▶ Two triangular bandages
▶ Get victim to the hospital	▶ Soft padding

SIGNS AND SYMPTOMS
▶ Pain and tenderness
▶ Victim attempts to relieve pain by supporting the elbow and not moving the arm
▶ Swelling or deformity at site of injury

1 Support arm

● Help the victim to position her arm on the injured side so that her fingertips rest on the uninjured collarbone.
● Ask her to support the affected arm at the elbow.

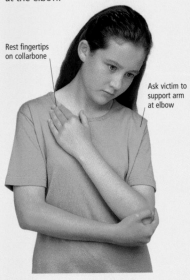

Rest fingertips on collarbone

Ask victim to support arm at elbow

2 Put arm in sling

● Put the arm in an elevation sling (p.29), being careful to move the arm as little as possible as you do so.

3 Position soft padding

● Place soft padding, such as a folded towel, between the victim's upper arm and chest to make her more comfortable.

4 Secure arm to chest

● Secure the arm to the victim's chest by tying a broad-fold bandage (p.27) over the sling and around her body.
● Check circulation in the thumb (see Roller bandages p.26).

Check circulation in thumb

5 Get victim to a hospital

✚ TAKE OR SEND VICTIM TO THE HOSPITAL

Arm injury

A break can occur anywhere along the upper arm or forearm and may involve the elbow or wrist joint.

SIGNS AND SYMPTOMS
▶ Pain and tenderness
▶ Reluctance to move injured arm
▶ Deformity, swelling, and bruising

Your aims	You will need
▶ Immobilize arm ▶ Get victim to the hospital	▶ Padding ▶ Two triangular bandages

1 Support arm

● If possible, gently bend the victim's arm at the elbow so that her arm is positioned across her body. Ask her to support her elbow with her other hand.
● Place padding, such as a folded towel, between the site of the break and the body.

2 Put arm in sling

● Put the arm in an arm sling (p.28).
● For extra support, secure the victim's arm to her body with a broad-fold bandage (p.27), making sure you avoid the site of the break.

3 Get victim to a hospital

✚ TAKE OR SEND VICTIM TO THE HOSPITAL

WARNING
▶ If the victim is unable to bend her arm, do not force it. Help her to lie down and place padding, such as a towel, around the injured elbow.

✚ CALL 911 OR LOCAL EMS

Hand and finger injury

Broken bones in the hands or fingers are often caused by crushing. There may also be a wound, which may cause bleeding.

SIGNS AND SYMPTOMS
▶ Pain and tenderness
▶ Reluctance to move injured hand
▶ Deformity, swelling, and bruising

Your aims	You will need
▶ Immobilize and raise injured hand ▶ Get victim to the hospital	▶ Disposable gloves ▶ Sterile wound dressing ▶ Soft padding ▶ Two triangular bandages

1 Raise hand

● If there is any bleeding, put on disposable gloves, if available. Raise the hand to control any bleeding and reduce swelling. If you can, remove any rings.

2 Support arm in sling

● If the hand or finger is bleeding, put a sterile wound dressing on it and place soft padding, such as cotton wool, around the hand.
● Support the arm in an elevation sling (p.29), securing it with a broad-fold bandage (p.27).

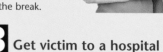

Support arm in elevation sling

3 Get victim to a hospital

✚ TAKE OR SEND VICTIM TO THE HOSPITAL

Rib injury

Broken ribs are held in place naturally because they are attached to the ribcage. To relieve the pain of a broken rib, support the arm on the affected side.

SIGNS AND SYMPTOMS
▶ Sharp pain in side, worsened by taking deep breaths, coughing, or movement
▶ Tenderness around affected ribs
▶ Crackling sound

Your aims	You will need
▶ Support victim's chest	▶ Two triangular bandages
▶ Get victim to the hospital	

1 Put arm in sling

● Make sure the victim is in a comfortable position, preferably sitting down.
● Support the arm in an arm sling (p.28).
● If necessary, secure the arm with a broad-fold bandage (p.27).

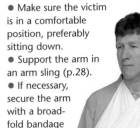

Support arm in sling

2 Get victim to a hospital

✚ TAKE OR SEND VICTIM TO THE HOSPITAL

WARNING
▶ If several ribs are damaged, the victim's breathing may be badly affected. Lean the victim toward his injured side with his head and shoulders well supported and his knees bent.

✚ CALL 911 OR LOCAL EMS

Pelvic injury

Treat a suspected fractured pelvis with great care because there may also be injuries to organs with possible internal bleeding.

SIGNS AND SYMPTOMS
▶ Pain, swelling, and inability to walk
▶ Desire to pass urine, which may be bloodstained
▶ Possible internal bleeding and shock

Your aims	You will need
▶ Relieve shock	▶ Padding
▶ Get victim to the hospital	▶ Blanket
	▶ Notepad and pen

1 Help victim lie down

● Help the victim on to his back with his legs straight or knees slightly bent.
● Put some padding, such as a cushion or rolled-up coat, under his knees for support.

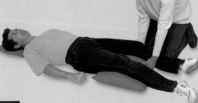

2 Treat for shock

● If necessary, treat the victim for shock (p.61).
● Reassure him and keep him warm.
● Do not allow him to eat or drink.

✚ CALL 911 OR LOCAL EMS

3 Monitor victim

● Monitor and record the victim's vital signs—level of response, pulse, and breathing (pp.20–1)—regularly until medical help arrives.

Spinal injury

Back injuries can be serious because they may affect the spinal cord, which contains the nerves that control many of the body's functions. A damaged spinal cord can result in paralysis of the body below the injured area. Always suspect a spinal injury if the victim has fallen awkwardly, especially from a height, and particularly if the victim has a head injury or is experiencing any loss of feeling or movement. Back injuries can be made worse by incorrect handling. Treat a conscious victim as described below. For an unconscious victim, see opposite.

Your aims	You will need
▶ Prevent further injury	▶ Coats/towels
▶ Get victim to the hospital urgently	▶ Blanket
	▶ Notepad and pen

SIGNS AND SYMPTOMS
▶ Tenderness around back
▶ Shooting pains or "electric shocks" in limbs and/ or trunk
▶ Inability to feel or move legs if injury is in lower back
▶ Inability to move any limb at all if injury is at neck level

1 Keep victim still

● Advise the victim not to move.
● Kneeling behind the victim's head, place your hands on either side of the head to support it with the head, neck, and spine aligned.

2 Support head, neck, and shoulders

● Use rolled-up coats or towels to protect and support the victim's head, neck, and shoulders.
● Cover the victim with a blanket.

✚ **CALL 911 OR LOCAL EMS**

Place rolled towels around head and shoulders

IMPORTANT
▶ Do not move the victim unless you believe his life is in danger.

Leave a gap between fingers and thumb so that victim can hear you

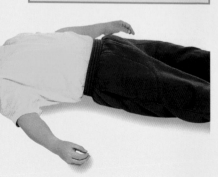

For an unconscious victim

- Kneel behind the victim's head and place your hands on either side of the head to support it with the head, neck, and spine aligned. Do not use immobilization devices.
- Ask a bystander to
✚ **CALL 911 OR LOCAL EMS**
- Open the victim's airway using the jaw-thrust method. Position your hands on either side of his face with your fingertips at the angles of his jaw. Gently lift his jaw forward with your fingers, without tilting his head back.

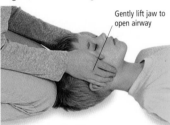

Gently lift jaw to open airway

- Check the victim's breathing (p.37 adults; p.46 children; p.50 infants). If he is breathing, support his head.
- If you need to leave the victim to call an ambulance or you are unable to keep the victim's airway open using the jaw thrust, put him into the adapted recovery position (p.39). Extend the arm nearest you above his head, and roll him toward you, keeping his head and trunk aligned, until his head rests on the extended arm.
- If the victim is not breathing, begin resuscitation (pp.36–52).
- If the victim is breathing, monitor and record his vital signs (pp.20–1) regularly until help arrives.

Leg injury

A broken leg is a serious injury. The thighbone has a rich blood supply and a break can cause severe internal bleeding. The shinbone lies just below the skin and, if broken, it may stick through the skin (p.104), making it susceptible to infection.

SIGNS AND SYMPTOMS
▶ Pain, swelling, and loss of movement
▶ Shock may develop
▶ Open wound with broken bone visible
▶ Injured leg may appear shortened
▶ Foot, and possibly knee, turned sideways

Your aims	You will need
▶ Support injured leg ▶ Get victim to the hospital urgently	▶ Sterile wound dressing

1 Support leg

- Help the victim to lie down carefully.
- Gently steady and support the leg with your hands at the joints above and below the site of the break.

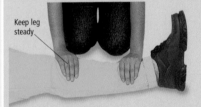

Keep leg steady

2 Treat wounds

- Cover any wounds with a sterile wound dressing (p.24).
✚ **CALL 911 OR LOCAL EMS**

3 Treat for shock

- Continue to support the leg to prevent any movement until the ambulance arrives. If necessary, treat for shock (p.61).

Ankle injury

A sprained ankle is the result of the ligaments that hold the bones together at the joints becoming stretched or torn (p.105). This injury is usually very painful and the symptoms can easily be mistaken for a broken bone (p.104). An ankle strain occurs when the muscles and tendons are torn by a sudden movement or violent contraction. Both injuries frequently take place during sporting activities.

Your aims	**You will need**
▶ Reduce swelling and pain	▶ Cold compress
▶ Get victim to the hospital if necessary or seek medical help	▶ Cotton padding
	▶ Roller bandage

SIGNS AND SYMPTOMS
▶ Swelling
▶ Pain and tenderness
▶ Inability to move ankle or stand on affected limb
▶ Gradual bruising

IMPORTANT
▶ Follow the RICE procedure if you suspect the victim has a sprain or a strain:

R	**I**	**C**	**E**
Rest	Ice	Compress	Elevate

▶ If you suspect the victim has a serious injury, for example he is in great pain and unable to move the affected foot,

➕**TAKE OR SEND VICTIM TO THE HOSPITAL**

1 Apply cold compress

● Help the victim to sit or lie down.
● Support the ankle in a comfortable position, such as on your knee.
● If the injury has just occurred, cool the ankle by applying a cold compress (p.25) for 10 minutes and then reassess the injury. Reapply a cold compress at 10-minute intervals for up to 30 minutes if necessary.

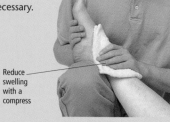

Reduce swelling with a compress

2 Bandage around ankle

● Place cotton padding around the ankle and press gently.
● Secure the padding with a roller bandage, leaving the toes exposed (p.26).
● Check the circulation in the toes (p.26) every 10 minutes.

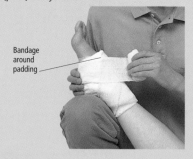

Bandage around padding

3 Raise limb

● Raise and support the injured limb to reduce the flow of blood to the injury, thereby reducing bruising.
● If the injury appears to be minor, advise the victim to rest and to seek medical help, if necessary.

Knee injury

It can be difficult to tell whether a person has a broken kneecap or has damaged cartilage or a ligament. If you are in any doubt, treat the injury as described below. The kneecap can be broken by a direct blow or split by a violent pull from the thigh muscles attached to it.

SIGNS AND SYMPTOMS
▶ Extreme pain
▶ Swelling

Your aim	You will need
▶ Get victim to the hospital urgently	▶ Pillows/coats ▶ Cotton padding ▶ Roller bandage

1 Support leg

● Help the victim to lie down.
● Steady and support her leg in a comfortable position.
● Place padding such as a pillow under her knee and rolled coats and/or pillows around her leg.

2 Bandage knee

● Wrap cotton padding around the knee.
● Secure the padding gently with a roller bandage (p.26).
✚ **CALL 911 OR LOCAL EMS**

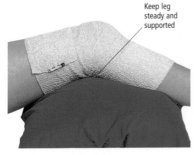

Keep leg steady and supported

Cramp

This pain can occur suddenly and is usually caused by a tightening, or contraction, of a single muscle or a group of muscles. Cramp can normally be relieved by stretching the affected muscles.

Your aim
▶ Relieve pain

In the hand

● Straighten the victim's bent fingers by gently stretching them backward.
● Massage the hand to relieve the cramp still further.

In the foot

● Straighten the victim's bent toes by gently pushing them upward.
● Help the victim to stand on the ball of her foot.

In the calf

● Straighten the victim's knee and pull the foot up towards the shin as far as possible.
● Gently massage the calf muscles.

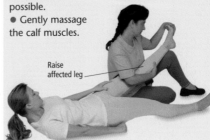

Raise affected leg

In the back of the thigh

● Straighten the victim's knee by pulling the leg up and forward, and gently, but firmly, press the knee down.

IMPORTANT
▶ Cramp may occur if a person has been sweating heavily. To relieve this, give the victim plenty of water to drink.

Test yourself

Now that you have read and studied the chapter on first-aid treatments for
bone, joint, and muscle injuries, see if you can answer the questions below.
Check your answers against the correct ones on page 144.

1 Which of the following should be your priorities when looking after a victim with a broken leg?
a Immobilize the leg .... ☐
b Reduce the swelling by cooling with water .... ☐
c Encourage the victim to try standing on the leg .... ☐
d Watch for shock .... ☐

2 What is an open break?
....
....

3 What is the risk with an open break that is not present with a closed break?
....
....

4 If you suspect that a victim has a broken bone, why should you not give him anything to eat, drink, or smoke?
....
....

5 What is the difference between a sprain and a strain?
....
....
....

6 How is a collarbone usually broken?
....
....

7 What are the signs and symptoms that might make you suspect that a victim's forearm is broken?
....
....
....

8 What are the likely complications if a victim has a pelvic injury?
....
....

9 What is your most important priority when dealing with a victim who has a suspected broken bone?
....
....
....

10 What do the letters R I C E stand for?
R ....
I ....
C ....
E ....

11 For how long should you leave a cold compress on an ankle injury?
....
....
....
....
....

12 How would you relieve cramp in a calf muscle?
....
....

7 Poisoning, bites, and stings

This chapter begins by explaining what to do if you suspect that someone has swallowed a poison. The effects of a poison vary considerably depending on what it is and how much is consumed. Poisoning is usually nonintentional and can be caused by exposure to toxic substances or eating or drinking them. It can also be caused by alcohol or drugs.

First-aid treatments for insect stings, which can be serious if a victim is allergic to the sting, and snake bites, which require prompt attention to prevent venom (poison) from spreading around the body, are also covered. Finally, the chapter sets out how to deal with animal bites, which always require medical attention because they may carry a risk of rabies and tetanus infections.

Use the questionnaire on page 122 to test your understanding of first aid for poisoning, bites, and stings.

IMPORTANT
POISON CONTROL CENTER
800 222 1222

Contents

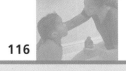

Dealing with poisoning

Poisons are substances that can cause temporary or permanent damage to the body if taken in large enough quantities. Poisons can be swallowed, absorbed or injected through the skin, splashed into the eyes, or breathed in through the lungs. The effects vary according to the poison and how it has been taken. Try to find out what was taken and how much—if the victim is conscious, ask what happened as soon as possible, as she may lose consciousness. If there are bystanders, ask them too.

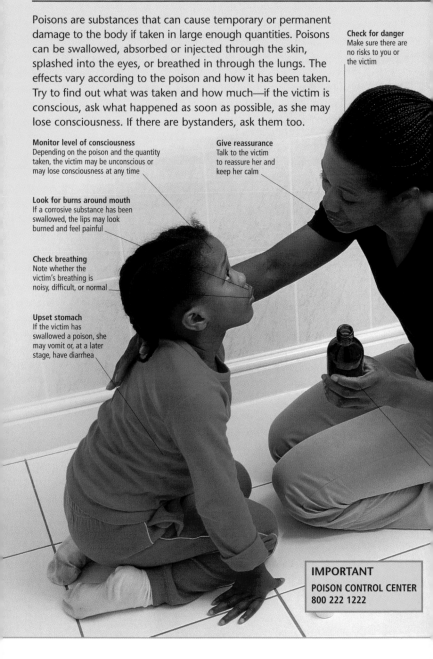

Check for danger
Make sure there are no risks to you or the victim

Monitor level of consciousness
Depending on the poison and the quantity taken, the victim may be unconscious or may lose consciousness at any time

Give reassurance
Talk to the victim to reassure her and keep her calm

Look for burns around mouth
If a corrosive substance has been swallowed, the lips may look burned and feel painful

Check breathing
Note whether the victim's breathing is noisy, difficult, or normal

Upset stomach
If the victim has swallowed a poison, she may vomit or, at a later stage, have diarrhea

IMPORTANT

POISON CONTROL CENTER
800 222 1222

What you should do

Your aims
▶ Identify poison
▶ Get victim to the hospital urgently
▶ Monitor victim

IMPORTANT
▶ Take care not to get any of the chemical on yourself. If you do (see Chemical burns p.81).
▶ Do not give the victim sips of milk or water.
▶ Do not try to make the vcitim vomit—anything that burns going down will burn again coming back up.
▶ Do not leave the victim alone unless you have to do so to call emergency services

1 Identify poison

● Look for any evidence of what the victim has taken: for example berries, medicine bottles, or pills.

2 Call Poison control center

● Call Poison control center and follow their advice.
● Do not give the victim anything to drink. Only give syrup of ipecac or activated charcoal if instructed to do so by the Posion control center.

3 Call 911 or local EMS

● Give dispatcher details of the poison and the amount the victim has taken.
● Keep any evidence of the poison taken for the emergency services.
● If the victim vomits, keep a sample for the emergency services.

4 Monitor victim

● Monitor and record the victim's vital signs—level of response, pulse, and breathing (pp.20–1)— regularly until help arrives.
● Pass on this information on to the emergency services.

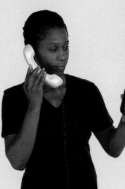

Give details of poison to emergency services dispatcher

Get a history
Ask the victim what she has taken. Look for clues nearby, such as containers, to identify the poison

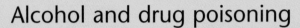

Alcohol and drug poisoning

Taken in excess, alcohol and drugs can seriously affect all physical and mental abilities. This can result in a victim falling and sustaining other injuries. If the victim is not fully conscious, there is a risk that he may vomit and inhale the vomit. Since alcohol and some drugs dilate the skin's blood vessels, the victim will lose heat and may develop hypothermia (p.86). If a victim smells of alcohol, excess alcohol may not be the only problem; check for other health problems, such as a stroke (p.96) or a heart attack (p.124).

Your aims	You will need
▶ Keep victim warm ▶ Check for other injuries and illnesses ▶ Get medical help if necessary	▶ Blanket/coat ▶ Notepad and pen

SIGNS AND SYMPTOMS

▶ Smell of alcohol
▶ Loss of coordination; confusion
▶ Flushed face
▶ Deep, noisy breathing

If victim becomes unconscious:
▶ Shallow breathing and weak pulse

If stimulant drugs have been taken:
▶ Raised body temperature and other symptoms of heatstroke (p.85)

1 Cover victim

● Help the victim to sit or lie down in a warm, comfortable place if possible.

● Cover him with a blanket or coat to help keep him warm.

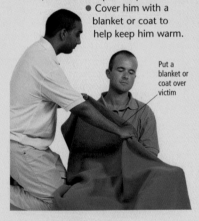

Put a blanket or coat over victim

2 Look for causes

● Look for empty containers that may indicate what the victim has taken.
● Keep a sample of any vomit in case it needs to be analyzed.
● Treat any injuries.

3 Monitor victim

● Get medical help if necessary.
● Monitor and record his vital signs (pp.20–1) regularly until help arrives.

Use of stimulant drugs

Stimulant drugs, such as ecstasy and cocaine, can lead to excitable, hyperactive behavior and possibly hallucinations, exhaustion, and overheating. For a victim needing first aid after taking a stimulant drug:

● Lower his body temperature by getting him to rest in a cool place (see Heatstroke p.85).
● Do not cover him with a blanket as this will increase his body temperature.

IMPORTANT

**POISON CONTROL CENTER
800 222 1222**

WARNING

▶ If the victim is unconscious,

✚ CALL 911 OR LOCAL EMS

Open the airway and check breathing. Put him in the recovery position if he is breathing. Be ready to begin resuscitation (pp.36–52).

Insect stings

The stings of a bee, wasp, or hornet are usually more alarming than dangerous, although multiple stings and stings in the mouth can be serious (below). Some people are allergic to stings (see Anaphylactic shock p.129) and will need urgent medical help.

Your aims	You will need
▶ Remove stinger	▶ Rigid piece of plastic, such as a credit card, to scrape off sting
▶ Relieve pain and swelling	
▶ Identify insect if possible	▶ Ice pack
▶ Get medical help if necessary	For stings in mouth or throat:
	▶ Ice cubes/cold water

SIGNS AND SYMPTOMS
▶ Pain at site of sting
▶ Slightly swollen, red, and sore skin

WARNING
▶ If the victim shows any signs of anaphylactic (allergic) shock (p.129),
✚ **CALL 911 OR LOCAL EMS**

1 Remove stinger

● If you can see the stinger, scrape it away carefully with your fingernail or a credit card.

Use credit card to scrape stinger away

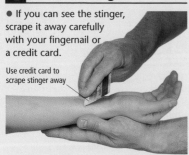

IMPORTANT
▶ Do not try to remove a stinger with tweezers because the sting may have a venom sac attached and you may squeeze more venom into the victim.

2 Apply ice pack

● Place an ice pack (p.25) on the affected area to reduce pain and swelling.

3 Rest injured part

● Keep the injured part in a comfortable position, preferably raised, until the pain and swelling ease.
● If you are concerned about continued pain and swelling,
✚ **GET MEDICAL HELP**

Stings in the mouth or throat

● A sting inside the mouth or throat is potentially very dangerous because the swelling it causes can obstruct the victim's airway. If you suspect a mouth or throat sting,
✚ **CALL 911 OR LOCAL EMS**
● If possible, give the victim an ice cube to suck or sips of cold water to reduce the swelling of the tissues lining the airway.

Get victim to take sips of water to reduce swelling

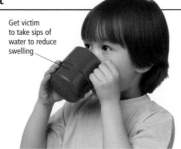

Snake bites

If a victim has been bitten by an elapid, or coral, snake (a poisonous snake with hollow, fixed fangs), loosely bandage the affected limb with an elastic bandage to prevent the venom spreading. Keep victim still and his heart above the level of the wound.

Your aims	You will need
▶ Stop venom spreading through body ▶ Reassure victim ▶ Get victim to the hospital urgently	▶ Soap and water ▶ Clean gauze swabs or other nonfluffy material ▶ Elastic roller bandage ▶ Towels/blanket ▶ Triangular bandage

SIGNS AND SYMPTOMS
▶ One or two small puncture marks
▶ Pain, redness, and possible swelling
▶ Nausea and vomiting
▶ Disturbed vision
▶ Sweating

WARNING
▶ Do not try to suck out the venom.
▶ If the victim becomes unconscious, open the airway and check breathing. Put her in the recovery position if she is breathing. Be ready to begin resuscitation if necessary (pp.36–52).

1 Help victim lie down

● Help the victim to lie down and tell her to keep still to slow down the spread of venom in the body.
● Reassure her.

2 Call 911 or local EMS

● Call the emergency services. If you can, describe the snake to the dispatcher so that the hospital knows which antivenom to give the victim.

3 Clean wound

● If possible, wash around the wound with soap and water.
● Pat the area dry with clean gauze swabs or other nonfluffy material.
● Wrap a roller bandage around the limb above the wound. Do not cover the bite.

4 Keep injured part still

● Place padding, such as rolled towels or blankets, around the injured area. Keep the padding in place with a triangular bandage (p.27).
● If a leg has been bitten, tie both legs together with broad-fold bandages.

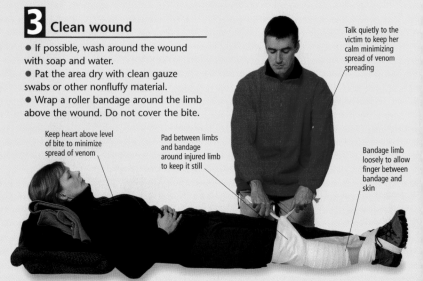

Talk quietly to the victim to keep her calm minimizing spread of venom spreading

Keep heart above level of bite to minimize spread of venom

Pad between limbs and bandage around injured limb to keep it still

Bandage limb loosely to allow finger between bandage and skin

Animal bites

Sharp teeth make deep wounds so animal bites can be serious. Prompt first aid is needed if the skin is broken to prevent infection. Animal bites carry the risk of tetanus infection or, more seriously, rabies, if the bite occurred in an affected area.

Your aims	You will need
▶ Control bleeding	▶ Disposable gloves
▶ Prevent infection	▶ Soap and water
▶ Get medical help if necessary	▶ Clean gauze swabs
	▶ Adhesive bandage or sterile wound dressing

IMPORTANT
▶ If there is a possibility of rabies, take or send the victim to the hospital immediately.
▶ Seek medical help if the victim has never had a tetanus injection, does not know when he was last injected or how many injections he has had, or it is more than 10 years since his last tetanus injection (p.62).

1 Press on wound

● Put on disposable gloves if available.
● If the wound is bleeding, press on the wound and raise the limb.

2 Clean and cover wound

● Wash the wound thoroughly with soap and water.
● Pat the wound dry with clean gauze swabs.
● Cover the wound with an adhesive bandage or sterile dressing.

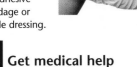

3 Get medical help

● If the wound is large or deep, take or send the victim to the hospital.

Marine injuries

Certain marine animals, such as corals and sea anemones, have painful stings that can be relieved with an ice pack. More serious injuries can be caused by tropical jellyfish stings and embedded spines from animals such as sea urchins and weever fish.

Your aims	You will need
▶ Reduce swelling	▶ Ice pack
▶ Get victim to the hospital if necessary	For a tropical jellyfish sting:
	▶ Vinegar or sea water
	▶ Roller bandage
	For an embedded spine:
	▶ Hot water

1 Help victim sit or lie down

● Get the victim to sit or lie down.
● Reassure the victim.

2 Apply ice pack

● Place an ice pack (p.25) on the affected area for 10 minutes.

IMPORTANT
▶ If the injury is severe or if the victim suffers a serious reaction to the sting,
✚ **CALL 911 OR LOCAL EMS**

For a tropical jellyfish sting

● Pour lots of vinegar or ocean water over the wound.
● Lightly cover the wound with a roller bandage.
✚ **CALL 911 OR LOCAL EMS**

For an embedded spine

● Soak the injured part in water as hot as the victim can bear for half an hour.
● Take or send the victim to the hospital to have the spine removed.

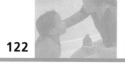

Test yourself

Now that you have read and studied the chapter on first-aid treatments for poisoning, bites, and stings, see if you can answer the questions below. Check your answers against the correct ones on page 144.

1 What are your aims when dealing with poisoning and what number should you call first?
....
....

2 If you need to give rescue breaths to an unconscious poisoned victim who has chemicals around his mouth, what should you do?
....
....

3 Which of the following are signs or symptoms of alcohol poisoning?
a Smell of alcohol on victim .... ☐
b Loss of coordination .... ☐
c Confusion..................................... ☐
d Flushed face .... ☐
e Deep, noisy breathing .... ☐
f Loss of consciousness...................... ☐

4 Why should you keep a victim with alcohol poisoning warm?
....
....

5 What is your priority when dealing with a victim who has taken stimulant drugs?
....
....

6 What is the best way to remove an insect sting?
....
....

7 Why should you not use tweezers to remove an insect sting?
....
....

8 Why is an insect sting in the mouth or throat particularly dangerous?
....
....

9 List three things to do to stop the spread of snake venom after a bite.
1...
2...
3...

10 What infections do animal bites carry the risk of?
....
....

11 What first aid would you give for a sea anemone sting?
....
....
....

12 What first aid would you give for a tropical jellyfish sting?
....
....
....

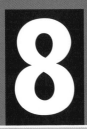

8 Medical problems and emergencies

This chapter covers a wide range of medical problems and emergencies that can affect a victim. It begins by explaining how to deal with someone who is having a heart attack. This is a life-threatening condition and every first aider needs to be aware of the risk that the heart may stop beating.

There are first-aid procedures for serious disorders that require urgent medical help, such as a diabetic emergency and anaphylactic shock. However, this chapter also deals with minor illnesses and disorders, such as headache, sore throat, and fever. While these are usually no cause for concern, it is important to be aware that they can be symptoms of a serious illness, such as meningitis.

Use the questionnaire on page 139 to test your understanding of first aid for medical problems and emergencies.

Contents

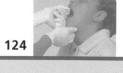

Dealing with a heart attack

A heart attack is caused by a blockage, usually a blood clot, that forms in an artery carrying blood to part of the heart muscle. This blockage is known as coronary thrombosis and its effects depend on how much of the heart muscle is damaged. The main risk of a heart attack is that the heart will go into an abnormal rhythm—ventricular fibrillation—and stop beating (cardiac arrest). If you suspect a heart attack, encourage the victim to rest and arrange for him to be taken to hospital as soon as possible.

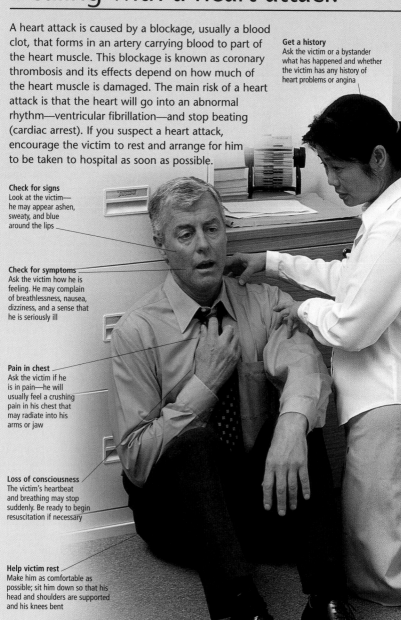

Get a history
Ask the victim or a bystander what has happened and whether the victim has any history of heart problems or angina

Check for signs
Look at the victim—he may appear ashen, sweaty, and blue around the lips

Check for symptoms
Ask the victim how he is feeling. He may complain of breathlessness, nausea, dizziness, and a sense that he is seriously ill

Pain in chest
Ask the victim if he is in pain—he will usually feel a crushing pain in his chest that may radiate into his arms or jaw

Loss of consciousness
The victim's heartbeat and breathing may stop suddenly. Be ready to begin resuscitation if necessary

Help victim rest
Make him as comfortable as possible; sit him down so that his head and shoulders are supported and his knees bent

WARNING
▶ If the victim becomes unconscious,

✚ **CALL 911 OR LOCAL EMS,**

Be ready to begin resuscitation (pp.36–52).

Give reasssurance
Tell the victim that you will call 911 or your local EMS and help him to take any medication

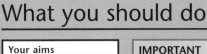

What you should do

Your aims
▶ Encourage victim to rest
▶ Get victim to hospital urgently

IMPORTANT
▶ Do not leave the victim alone unless you have to do so in order to get help.
▶ Do not allow the victim to eat, drink, or smoke.

1 Help victim sit down

● Help the victim to sit down, making him as comfortable as possible.
● Ideally, help him lean back against a wall or chair so that his head and shoulders are supported and his knees are bent.

2 Call 911 or local EMS

● Call the emergency services immediately.
● Tell the dispatcher that you suspect the victim has had a heart attack.

3 Give aspirin

● If the victim is conscious, give him a 300mg aspirin pill to chew slowly.

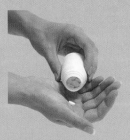

4 Give any other medication

● If the victim has any other medication, such as an aerosol for angina, help him to take it.

5 Regularly check victim

● Monitor and record the victim's vital signs—level of response, pulse, and breathing (pp.20–1)—regularly until help arrives. Watch for deterioration.

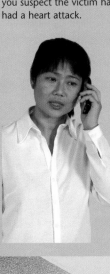

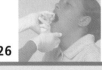

Angina

A person with angina feels a tight pain in the chest due to a narrowing of the arteries, resulting in an inadequate supply of oxygen and nutrients to the heart muscle. It is usually brought on by exercise and relieved by rest, but it may also be caused by anything that increases the activity of the heart, such as extreme emotion or excitement.

Your aims	You will need
▶ Help victim to rest to ease strain on heart ▶ Help victim take his own medication ▶ Get medical help if necessary	▶ Casualty's own medication

SIGNS AND SYMPTOMS
▶ Pain in middle of chest, sometimes spreading to jaw or arms
▶ Pain that eases with rest
▶ Breathlessness
▶ Anxiety

1 Get victim to rest

- Help the victim to sit down.
- Make sure he feels comfortable.
- Reassure him.

2 Help victim take medication

- If necessary, help the victim to find his medication.
- Help him to correctly identify his medication.
- Help him to take his medication.

3 Get medical help

- Advise the victim to seek medical help if he is still anxious after the angina has gone away.

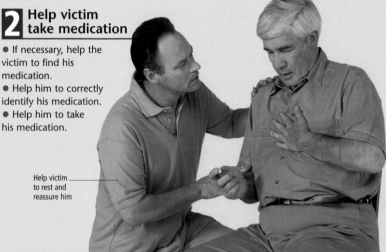

Help victim to rest and reassure him

WARNING
▶ If the pain does not ease after the victim has rested and taken medication or if the angina returns, suspect a heart attack and

✚ **CALL 911 OR LOCAL EMS**

▶ Treat as for a heart attack (p.124) and be ready to begin resuscitation if necessary (pp.36–52).
▶ If the victim becomes unconscious, open the airway and check breathing. Put him in the recovery position if he is breathing. Be ready to begin resuscitation if necessary (pp.36–52).

Diabetic emergency

A person who is diabetic is unable to produce the right amounts of insulin in the body—insulin is a chemical that controls how much sugar there is in the blood. Too much insulin results in abnormally low levels of sugar in the blood, a condition known as hypoglycemia. Too little insulin leads to a buildup of sugar in the blood, a condition known as hyperglycemia. Both conditions can be serious.

Hypoglycemia (low sugar)

Your aims	You will need
▶ Increase sugar content in blood ▶ Get medical help	▶ Sugary drink or sweet food ▶ Notepad and pen

SIGNS AND SYMPTOMS
▶ MedicAlert bracelet/syringe pen/tablets or gel
▶ Sweating; cold, clammy, and pale skin
▶ Strong pulse and heart palpitations
▶ Hunger, weakness, and faintness
▶ Confusion and low level of response
▶ Shallow breathing

1 Give sugary drink or food

● Help the victim to sit down. Give him a sugary drink or something sweet to eat.

2 Advise victim to rest

● If the victim starts to feel better, give him more food or drink.
● Advise him to rest and to see his doctor as soon as possible.

Hyperglycemia (high sugar)

Your aim	You will need
▶ Get victim to the hospital urgently	▶ Notepad and pen

SIGNS AND SYMPTOMS
▶ Dry skin
▶ Deep, heavy breathing; fast pulse
▶ Breath smelling of acetone (acetone smells like nail varnish remover or pear drops)
▶ Extreme thirst
▶ Casualty may become dazed and confused and may eventually lose consciousness

1 Call 911 or local EMS

● If you suspect that the victim is suffering from hyperglycemia, call the emergency services immediately.

2 Monitor victim

● Monitor and record his vital signs— level of response, breathing, and pulse (pp.20–1)—regularly until help arrives.

IMPORTANT
▶ It can be difficult to tell whether a victim is suffering from hypoglycemia or hyperglycemia. If the victim appears unwell and you know that he has diabetes, give him something sugary to drink. This will quickly correct hypoglycemia and cause little harm if he is suffering from hyperglycemia.

For an unconscious victim with hypo- or hyperglycemia

✚ CALL 911 OR LOCAL EMS
● Open the victim's airway and check breathing. Put him in the recovery position if he is breathing. Be ready to begin resuscitation (pp.36–52).

● Monitor and record the victim's vital signs—level of response, breathing, and pulse (pp.20–1)—regularly until help arrives.

Allergy

An allergy occurs when the body reacts to a substance, such as a food, chemical, drug, or plant pollen, that for most people is usually harmless. Symptoms of an allergy vary depending on the substance that triggers it. The most common ones include breathing difficulties, such as asthma (p.130), skin rashes, abdominal pain (p.138), or vomiting and diarrhea (p.138). Some people may experience very severe allergic reactions that can be life threatening (see Anaphylactic shock opposite).

Your aims	You will need
▶ Check severity of allergy	▶ Drinking water
▶ Treat mild symptoms	▶ Casualty's own medication
▶ Get medical help	

SIGNS AND SYMPTOMS
▶ Itchy red rash or raised areas of skin
▶ Breathing difficulties
▶ Abdominal pain
▶ Vomiting and diarrhea

1 Check symptoms

● Find out how severe the victim's symptoms are.
● Ask her if she has any known allergies.

2 Treat mild symptoms

● If the victim has vomited, give her water to sip.
● Make her comfortable.
● Help the victim take any medication that she might already have for her allergy.

3 Get medical help

● Advise victim to seek medical help.

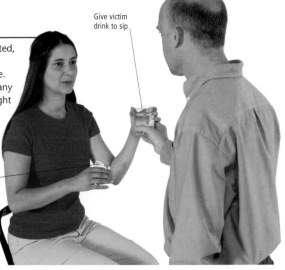

Give victim drink to sip

Help victim take prescribed allergy medication

IMPORTANT

▶ If the allergic reaction worsens, ask the victim if she has any medication, such as an autoinjector, to treat anaphylactic shock (opposite). Be prepared to help her use the autoinjector.

▶ If you are still concerned about the victim's condition or if she finds it difficult to breathe or appears distressed,

✚ CALL 911 OR LOCAL EMS

Anaphylactic (allergic) shock

This is a severe allergic reaction that may occur after an insect sting or after eating certain foods, such as peanuts. The reaction can be fast; the victim may find it hard to breathe and will need urgent medical help as she may lose consciousness. Some people know they suffer from this condition and carry epinephrine with them—often in the form of a preloaded syringe called an autoinjector. Help the victim to administer the medication or, if you are trained to do so, administer it yourself.

Your aim
▶ Get victim to the hospital urgently

1 Call 911 or local EMS

● Call the emergency services; tell the dispatcher that you suspect anaphylaxis.

2 Ease breathing

● Help the victim into a sitting position to ease any breathing difficulties.
● Help her to find and use any prescribed medication, such as an autoinjector.
● If the victim is unable to use her autoinjector and you have been trained in its use, give it to her yourself.

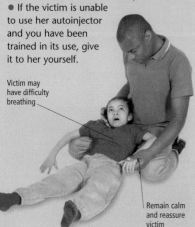

Victim may have difficulty breathing

Remain calm and reassure victim

3 Provide information

● Give emergency service personnel any information that will help identify the cause of the anaphylactic reaction.

SIGNS AND SYMPTOMS
▶ Anxiety
▶ Breathing difficulties and wheezing
▶ Blotchy, red skin
▶ Swollen face and neck; puffy eyes
▶ Fast pulse

WARNING
▶ If the victim becomes unconscious,
✚ **CALL 911 OR LOCAL EMS**
Open the airway and check breathing. Be ready to begin resuscitation if necessary (pp.36–52).

Using autoinjectors

A victim with a known allergy may have her own medication to take in case of an attack. This usually takes the form of a syringe or autoinjector of epinephrine.
To give it to her:
● Hold the autoinjector with your fingers and remove the protective cap.
● Holding the autoinjector with your fist, place the tip firmly against the victim's thigh to release the medication. Rub the injection site.

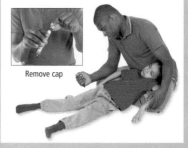

Remove cap

Asthma

An asthma attack occurs when a person's airways narrow, causing wheezing and breathing difficulties. A stimulus, such as dust, can trigger an attack or asthma may occur for no apparent reason. Most asthmatics use a reliever inhaler to treat themselves. Reassuring the victim may help to make him feel less anxious and ease an attack.

Your aims
▸ Help victim breathe more easily
▸ Get medical help if necessary

SIGNS AND SYMPTOMS
▸ Difficulty breathing, especially breathing out
▸ Wheezy cough
▸ Anxiety and signs of distress
▸ Bluish tinge to lips and face
▸ Tiredness
▸ Difficulty talking

---

1 Reassure victim

● Remain calm and reassure the victim.
● Help her to find and use a reliever inhaler, if she has one; using it should help her to breathe more easily. Tell her to try to breathe slowly and deeply.

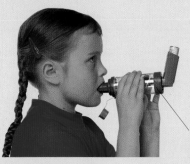

Use a reliever inhaler to make breathing easier

3 Call 911 or local EMS

● It is necessary to call the emergency services if: the attack is severe and the victim has difficulty talking; her breathing has not improved five minutes after using the inhaler; she is becoming exhausted; or if this is her first attack.
● Help the victim to use her inhaler every five to 10 minutes while you wait for the help and continue to reassure her.

2 Make victim comfortable

● Help the victim to relax in the position that she finds most comfortable—this will usually be sitting slightly forward with the arms resting on a firm surface, such as the back of a chair.
● If the attack has not passed within three minutes, ask the victim to take another dose of her inhaler.
● If you are concerned, advise the victim to seek medical advice.

IMPORTANT
▸ Do not force a victim to lie down during an asthma attack.
▸ Do not ask the victim unnecessary questions; answering you will make her even more breathless.

WARNING
▸ If the victim loses consciousness,
✚ **CALL 911 OR LOCAL EMS**

Open the airway and check breathing. Put her in the recovery position if she is breathing. Be ready to begin resuscitation if necessary (pp.36–52).
▸ Monitor and record the victim's vital signs—level of response, pulse, and breathing (pp.20–1)—regularly until help arrives.

Croup

An attack of croup is caused when a young child's larynx and windpipe (trachea) become inflamed, making breathing difficult. The noise a child with croup makes may sound alarming, but the symptoms will usually pass quickly without causing the child any lasting damage. A child is more likely to suffer an attack of croup at night.

Your aims
▶ Comfort and support child
▶ Make breathing easier

SIGNS AND SYMPTOMS
▶ Distressed breathing
▶ Short, barking cough
▶ Whistling noise, especially when child breathes in
▶ Blue-gray skin (cyanosis) in severe cases

1 Comfort child

● Sit the child on your knee, make him feel secure, and reassure him.

2 Make steamy atmosphere

● To ease breathing, create a steamy atmosphere either in the bathroom by running the hot water tap in the bath or in the kitchen by boiling the kettle.
● Encourage the child to breathe in the steam.
● After his breathing eases, put the child back to bed.
● Create a steamy atmosphere in the bedroom, if possible, perhaps by hanging a wet towel over a hot radiator.

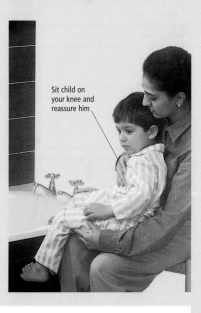

Sit child on your knee and reassure him

IMPORTANT
▶ If the croup is severe, persists, or you are worried,
✚ **CALL 911 OR LOCAL EMS**

Epiglottitis

This disorder is caused by the epiglottis—the small, flaplike structure in the back of the throat—becoming inflamed. It is a life-threatening condition because the swollen epiglottis may block the airway. It can affect children and adults.

The signs and symptoms of epiglottitis are:
● High temperature
● Distressed breathing
● Difficulty coughing
● Difficulty swallowing
● Whistling noise when breathing in and out
● The victim is obviously ill but sits upright.

If you suspect epiglottitis,
✚ **CALL 911 OR LOCAL EMS**
● Do not try to ease the breathing by putting your fingers down the throat; this may cause the muscles in the throat to go into spasm and quickly block the airway.

Object in the eye

The most common types of foreign object that get into the eyes are pieces of grit, dust, eyelashes, or small insects. Most of them are easily removed. However, you should not attempt to remove anything that sticks to the eye because this may cause damage.

Your aims	You will need
▶ Prevent injury to eye	▶ Jug of water or sterile
▶ Remove foreign object	eyewash
	▶ Bowl and towel
	▶ Moist gauze pad/clean handkerchief

SIGNS AND SYMPTOMS
▶ Pain or discomfort in eye; blurred vision
▶ Redness and watering of the eye

1 Help victim sit down

● Tell the victim not to rub her eye.
● Ask her to sit down in a chair facing a light and to lean back slightly.

2 Examine eye

● Stand behind the victim and ask her to look up.
● Supporting her chin, gently separate the eyelids and look for the foreign object.

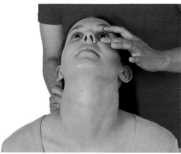

IMPORTANT
▶ Do not remove anything from the colored part of the eye or anything that is stuck in the eye. Instead, cover the eye with a sterile wound dressing and get the victim to the hospital.

WARNING
▶ If you are unable to remove the foreign object,
✚ **TAKE OR SEND VICTIM TO THE HOSPITAL**

3 Removing an object on eyelid or white of eye

● If you can see the object inside the eyelid or on the white of the eye, pour water or sterile eyewash into the inner corner of the eye to flush it out. Place a towel on the victim's shoulder and get her to hold a bowl to catch any drips.
● If this does not work, lift it off with a moist gauze pad or clean handkerchief.

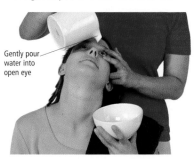

Gently pour water into open eye

4 Removing an object under upper eyelid

● If the particle is under the upper lid, ask the victim to look down, grasp her upper lid by the lashes, and draw it out and down over the lower lid.
● If the object is still there, bathe eye with water or eyewash and ask her to blink; the object should float off.

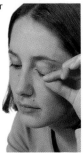

Object in the ear

Young children have a habit of putting objects such as beads into their ears; adults may leave cotton in theirs after cleaning them; and insects may fly or crawl into ears. A foreign object in the ear may cause temporary deafness or even damage the eardrum.

Your aims	**You will need**
▶ Reassure victim	For removing an insect:
▶ Prevent injury to ear	▶ Towel
▶ Remove foreign object	▶ Tepid water
	▶ Jug/glass

1 Examine ear

● Reassure the victim.
● Look into the ear to see what the foreign object is.

2 Tilt victim's head

● If the object is a bead or something similar, tilt the victim's head so that the affected ear is facing downward; the object may drop out.

> **WARNING**
> ▶ If the object does not fall out of the ear, do not try to dig it out with your fingers or any other instrument.
> ✚ **TAKE OR SEND VICTIM TO THE HOSPITAL**

Removing an insect

● If an insect is in the victim's ear, tell her to tilt her head to one side with the affected ear facing up.
● Place a towel over her shoulder and support her head with your hand.
● Gently pour tepid water from a jug or glass into the ear; the insect should float to the surface.
● If the insect does not float to the surface, take the victim to the hospital.

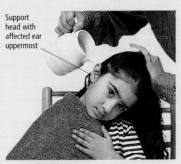

Support head with affected ear uppermost

Object in the nose

It is quite common for young children to push small objects up their noses. These may block the nose and cause an infection. If the object is sharp, it may damage the lining of the nose.

1 Reassure victim

● Try to keep the victim quiet and calm; tell him to breathe steadily through the mouth.
● Do not try to remove the foreign object, even if you can see it.

Your aims
▶ Reassure victim
▶ Get victim to the hospital

SIGNS AND SYMPTOMS
▶ Difficult or noisy breathing through nose
▶ Swelling of nose
▶ Smelly or bloodstained discharge from nose

2 Get victim to a hospital

● Take or send the victim to the hospital.

Toothache

Decay in a tooth is usually the cause of toothache, especially if the pain does not go away. Toothache is often made worse by hot or cold food or drink. If it is a throbbing pain, there may be an infection at the root of the tooth.

Your aims	You will need
▶ Relieve pain	▶ Hot-water bottle
▶ Advise victim to see a dental practitioner	▶ Towel
	▶ Cotton
	▶ Oil of cloves

1 Relieve pain

● An adult may take two acetaminophen tablets and a child may be given the recommended dose of acetaminophen elixir.

● Give the victim a hot-water bottle wrapped in a towel to hold against his cheek. Alternatively, give him a rolled-up plug of cotton soaked in oil of cloves to hold against the affected tooth.

Hold hot-water bottle wrapped in towel against cheek

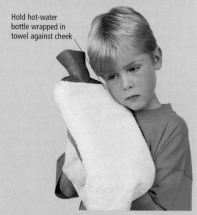

2 Get dental help

● Advise the victim to see his dental practitioner as soon as possible.

Earache

This common condition is caused by inflammation inside the ear, which is often a result of an infection linked to a cold, tonsillitis, or flu, especially in children. The victim's hearing may also be impaired, but this is usually temporary.

Your aims	You will need
▶ Relieve pain	▶ Hot-water bottle
▶ Get medical help	▶ Towel

1 Relieve pain

● An adult may take two acetaminophen tablets and a child may be given the recommended dose of acetaminophen elixir.

● Get the victim to hold a hot-water bottle wrapped in a towel against his ear.

Hold hot-water bottle wrapped in towel against ear

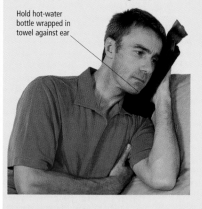

2 Get medical help

● Advise the victim to see his doctor if the earache persists.

IMPORTANT
▶ If there is any discharge from the ear, a fever, or marked hearing loss,

✚ **GET MEDICAL HELP**

Headache

A headache is usually caused by tiredness and tension, but it can accompany a feverish illness, such as flu, or be part of a migraine attack (right). A headache can also be an indication of something more serious, such as a stroke (p.96) or meningitis (p.137).

Your aim	You will need
▶ Relieve pain	▶ Cold compress

1 Make victim comfortable

● Help the victim to sit or lie down in a quiet place.

2 Apply cold compress

● Place a cold compress (p.25) on the victim's head.
● An adult may take two acetominophen tablets and a child may be given the recommended dose of acetominophen elixir.

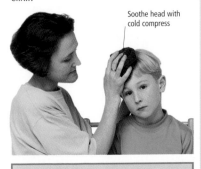

Soothe head with cold compress

IMPORTANT

✚ **CALL 911 OR LOCAL EMS**

If the pain:
▶ Develops suddenly
▶ Is severe and incapacitating
▶ Is recurrent or persistent
▶ Is accompanied by a stiff neck
▶ Follows a head injury
▶ Is accompanied by a dazed feeling.

Migraine

A migraine is usually an intense, throbbing headache on one side of the head. Before an attack the victim's vision may be disturbed. During an attack, the victim may have nausea and vomiting and find it hard to tolerate bright light. Attacks may be triggered by a number of causes, including certain foods, such as cheese or chocolate, an allergy, or tiredness.

Your aim
▶ Relieve pain

1 Relieve pain

● If the victim has her own medication, encourage her to take it.
● If an adult does not have medication, she may take two acetominophen tablets; a child may be given the recommended dose of acetominophen elixir.

2 Advise victim to sleep

● Get the victim to lie down in a cool, dark room and sleep for a few hours.

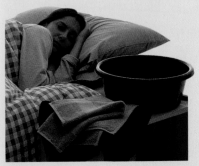

IMPORTANT

Get medical help if:
▶ It is the victim's first migraine attack
▶ Vomiting is severe
▶ Victim is concerned.

Sore throat

A sore throat may be the first sign of a cough or cold and will usually pass in a couple of days. It may also be caused by tonsillitis—a more serious condition—in which the tonsils at the back of the throat become infected with bacteria or viruses. The tonsils appear red and swollen, and ulcers or white spots of pus may also be visible. Swallowing may be difficult.

Your aims	You will need
▶ Relieve pain	▶ Cool drinks
▶ Get medical help if necessary	

1 Give water

● Give the victim plenty of cool drinks, particularly water, which will ease the pain and stop the throat becoming dry.
● An adult may take two acetaminophen tablets and a child may be given the recommended dose of acetaminophen elixir.

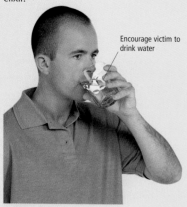

Encourage victim to drink water

2 Get medical help

● If the pain is severe and you suspect the victim has tonsillitis, advise him to see a doctor as soon as possible.

Fever

A fever is a body temperature that stays above the normal level of 98.6°F (37°C). It is usually a sign of an infection, either a local infection such as an abscess or a general infection such as chickenpox.

Your aims	You will need
▶ Bring down temperature	▶ Cool, damp flannel
▶ Get medical help if necessary	▶ Cool drinks

1 Bring down temperature

● Keep the victim comfortable and cool, preferably in bed.
● Gently wipe her forehead with a cool, damp flannel.
● Give plenty of cool, bland drinks.
● An adult may take two acetaminophen tablets and a child may be given the recommended dose of acetaminophen elixir.

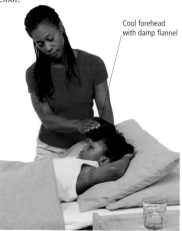

Cool forehead with damp flannel

2 Get medical help

● If the fever lasts for longer than 24 hours, the victim should see a doctor.

Meningitis

This serious illness, which can affect anyone regardless of age, needs prompt medical treatment. It is caused by a viral or bacterial inflammation of the coverings of the brain. There are many signs and symptoms—the most common are listed below—but they are not usually all present at the same time. Without immediate treatment, permanent disability such as deafness or brain damage may result; the illness can be fatal.

Your aims	You will need
▶ Get victim to the hospital urgently ▶ Reassure victim	▶ Cool, damp flannel

SIGNS AND SYMPTOMS

Illness starts with:
▶ Flulike illness
▶ High temperature
▶ Cold hands and feet, and limb pain
▶ Mottled skin

As infection develops:
▶ Headache
▶ Stiff neck (victim cannot touch chest with chin)
▶ Vomiting
▶ Sensitivity to bright light
▶ Increasing drowsiness
▶ Distinctive rash (see Identifying the rash below).

1 Call 911 or local EMS

● If you suspect meningitis, call the emergency services immediately.

2 Treat the fever and reassure victim

● Treat the fever (see opposite).
● Stay with the victim while you wait for the help to arrive.
● Keep him cool, quiet, and comfortable.

WARNING
▶ Do not wait for all the above signs and symptoms to be present before seeking medical help.

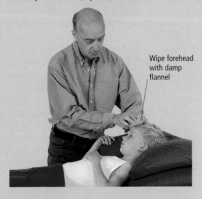

Wipe forehead with damp flannel

Identifying the rash

A meningitis rash is distinctive and has the following features:
● It does not fade when pressed.
● Small red or purple pinprick spots spread to look like fresh bruising.
● It may appear late in the course of the illness or it may not come at all.
● It is not so easy to see on dark skin.

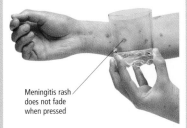

Meningitis rash does not fade when pressed

IMPORTANT
▶ When calling the emergency services, describe the symptoms and say that you suspect meningitis.
▶ Be prepared to insist on medical attention.
▶ If the victim is obviously unwell and his condition worsens, even if he has already been seen by a doctor, seek urgent medical attention again.

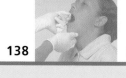

Abdominal pain

Pain in the abdomen usually indicates a relatively minor ailment such as food poisoning, but occasionally it may be a sign of a more serious condition such as appendicitis or a bowel obstruction.

Your aims	You will need
▶ Relieve pain	▶ Hot-water bottle
▶ Reassure victim	▶ Towel
▶ Get medical help if necessary	

1 Make victim comfortable

● Make the victim as comfortable as possible.
● Reassure her.
● Give her a hot-water bottle wrapped in a towel to hold against the abdomen.

Soothe pain with hot-water bottle wrapped in towel

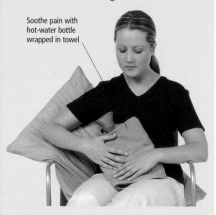

2 Get medical help

● See a doctor if the pain is severe, if the pain is accompanied by a fever and vomiting, or if you are concerned by the victim's condition.

Vomiting and diarrhea

These problems, which can occur together or separately, are usually the result of an irritated or infected digestive system. They may lead to dehydration, particularly if they happen at the same time, especially in infants and elderly people.

Your aims	You will need
▶ Reassure victim	▶ Bowl
▶ Restore body fluids	▶ Warm, damp cloth
▶ Get medical help if necessary	▶ Water

1 Make victim comfortable

● Reassure victim.
● Give her a bowl for vomit and a warm, damp cloth for wiping her face.

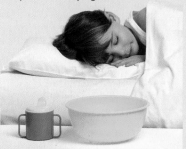

2 Give drinks

● When the vomiting subsides, give the victim plenty of clear fluids, such as water or nonfizzy drinks in frequent small sips, to restore lost body fluids.

3 Get medical help

● See a doctor if the vomiting or diarrhea does not stop or if you are concerned by the victim's condition.

Test yourself

Now that you have read and studied the chapter on first-aid treatments for medical problems and emergencies, see if you can answer the questions below. Check your answers against the correct ones on page 144.

1 What causes a heart attack?
....
....
....
....

2 What is the main risk associated with a heart attack?
....
....
....
....

3 Which of the following signs and symptoms indicate a heart attack?
a Blueness around lips .... □
b Nosebleed .... □
c Breathlessness .... □
d Blisters on the skin .... □
e Crushing pain in chest .... □
f Dizziness .... □

4 What are the priorities when treating a person known to have diabetes who is unwell but conscious?
....
....
....
....

5 What are the dangers to a victim of a severe allergic reaction?
....
....
....
....
....

6 What might a victim with a known severe allergy carry with him at all times?
....
....
....

7 In which of the following circumstances would you call an ambulance for a victim who is having an asthma attack?
a If the attack is severe and the victim has trouble speaking .... □
b If it is the victim's first attack of asthma .... □
c If the victim's breathing has not improved five minutes after using her inhaler .... □
d If the victim's breathing improves quickly after using her inhaler .... □
e If the victim is becoming exhausted ..... □

8 What is it most important to do when treating a high temperature (fever) and how would you do it?
....
....
....
....
....

9 If a victim has a fever, what other signs and symptoms indicate that he or she might have meningitis?
....
....
....
....
....

10 Name three problems that can be helped by holding a hot-water bottle against the affected part of the body?
1 ....
2 ....
3 ....

Index

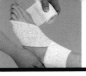

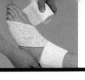

Acknowledgments

DORLING KINDERSLEY
Project manager Nigel Duffield
DTP Designer David McDonald
Production manager Sylvia La Greca Bertacchi

Produced for Dorling Kindersley by
COOLING BROWN

Creative Director Arthur Brown
Project Editor Jemima Dunne
Designer Peter Cooling

Cooling Brown would like to thank Evelynne Stoikou
and Sally Tynan for the models' make-up, and Hilary Bird
for compiling the index

Models Francesca Agati, Christine Appella, Angela Cameron,
Madelane Cameron, Scott Davis, Emma Forge, Jessica Forge,
Mark Ireland, Alastair King, Natalie King, Olivia King,
Crispin Lord, Philip Lord, Eric Lowes, Kincaid Malik-White,
Tony Mayne, Camilla Moore, Juliette Norsworthy,
Sagaren Pillay, Anna Pizzi, Eleanor Ridge, Sheila Tait,
Suki Tan, Peter Taylor, Jeremy Wallis, Tim Webster

Illustrator Patrick Mulrey

Photographers Trish Gant, Steve Gorton, Dave King,
Gary Ombler, Matthew Ward
All other images © Dorling Kindersley.
For further information see: **www.dkimages.com**

Test yourself: answers

Chapter 1 First-aid principles, page 30
1 Make sure that you are not in danger. 2 Call the emergency services and do not approach the scene of the incident. 3 The quietest ones because they may be unconscious. 4 Disposable gloves. 5 A specially designed yellow box used for the disposal of hypodermic needles and other sharp objects. 6 Dial 999 and ask for the relevant service (fire, ambulance, or police). 7 A = Alert; V = Voice; P = Pain; U = Unresponsive. 8 At the wrist (radial pulse), at the neck (carotid pulse), or in babies on the inside of the upper arm (brachial pulse). 9 a; c; d; and f. A blanket (b) and scissors (e) are useful additions but not basic requirements. 10 Because it will not slip and is easy to undo. Also, since it lies flat against the body it is more comfortable for the victim. 11 The ice will burn the skin. 12 Press the skin of the finger or toe until it turns pale and then watch for color to return. 13 Arm sling: to support an injured upper arm, forearm, or wrist and to immobilize an arm if there is a chest injury. Elevation sling: to support the arm in a raised position when a hand or forearm is injured and bleeding needs to be controlled; to support a broken hand; to reduce swelling in an injured arm; to support an arm in the event of a broken collarbone or rib.

Chapter 2 Life-saving techniques, page 56
1 Airway, breathing, and circulation. 2 Heart. 3 Open the airway; check breathing; put the victim in the recovery position; then call an ambulance. 4 One second 5 When giving rescue breaths, a face mask will prevent cross infection. 6 Cardiopulmonary resuscitation, which is a combination of rescue breathing and chest compressions. 7 Center of the chest. 8 For an adult, child, or infant, give two rescue breaths then 30 compressions. For a victim of any age, chest compressions should be given at a rate of 100 per minute. 9 A machine that restarts a heart that has an abnormal heart rhythm (known as ventricular fibrillation). 10 a; c; d; and f. 11 Abdominal thrusts.

Chapter 3 Wounds and bleeding, page 74
1 c; a; and then e. 2 Cover with a second dressing. If blood seeps through the second dressing, remove both and apply a new one. 3 Arteries; capillaries; veins. 4 Shock. 5 Rinse the wound, clean around it with a fresh swab or wipe, pick out any loose foreign matter, and cover with a adhesive dressing or sterile wound dressing. To prevent cross infection, you should also wear disposable gloves when treating the victim. 6 Level of response; pulse; and breathing. 7 To reduce blood flow to the bruise, thereby reducing swelling and pain. 8 Lean forward; pinch the soft part of the nose. 9 a or b. 10 A skull fracture. 11 Pinch the edges of the wound together around the embedded object.

Chapter 4 Environmental injuries, page 88
1 Cool the burn, prevent infection, treat any signs of shock, and get medical help. 2 Superficial burn; partial-thickness burn; full-thickness burn. 3 Fluid loss leading to shock. 4 Do not apply creams, sprays, ointments, or adhesive tape to the burn; do not touch the burned area; do not remove any clothing sticking to the burn. 5 Clean plastic bag, clean tea towel, clean sheet, or plastic wrap. 6 Damaged skin and/or soot around the mouth. 7 Cool for at least 10 minutes. If you cool a burn for too long, there is a risk of hypothermia. 8 At least 20 minutes to wash off all the chemical. 9 Break the victim's contact with the electricity. 10 Dehydration. 11 Signs and symptoms include loss of consciousness; very cold, pale skin; shivering; clumsiness; irritability; slurred speech; slow breathing; weak pulse; and lethargy. 12 To warm the affected part slowly and to get the victim to hospital.

Chapter 5 Disorders affecting consciousness, page 100
1 They can affect the victim's level of consciousness. 2 Bruising and/or bleeding of the scalp; concussion; compression; fracture to the skull; injury to the spine. 3 The victim's level of response deteriorates after a head injury. 4 The victim is dazed and confused, probably for a few minutes, before making a full recovery. 5 Open the victim's airway, check his breathing, and be ready to begin resuscitation if necessary. 6 b and c. 7 A brief loss of consciousness due to the reduced flow of blood to the brain. 8 c. 9 Protect the child from injury; cool him; call an ambulance. 10 Level of response; pulse; and breathing.

Chapter 6 Bone, joint, and muscle injuries, page 114
1 a and d. 2 An injury in which a bone is broken along with a break in the skin, sometimes with the bone protruding. 3 Infection. 4 The victim may later need a general anesthetic. 5 A sprain is a torn ligament (a fibrous band that holds bones together at a joint) and a strain is an overstretched muscle or tendon (a fibrous band that attaches a muscle to a bone). 6 As a result of an indirect force, for example from falling onto an outstretched hand. 7 Pain and tenderness; reluctance to move injured arm; deformity, swelling, and bruising. 8 Internal bleeding and shock. 9 Keep the affected part still to prevent broken bone ends causing further damage to blood vessels, tissues, or internal organs. 10 Rest; Ice; Compress; Elevate. 11 For 10 minutes and reassess the injury. Reapply at 10-minute intervals for up to 30 minutes if necessary. 12 Straighten the victim's knee and pull the foot up towards the shin as far as possible, and then gently massage the calf muscles.

Chapter 7 Poisoning, bites, and stings, page 122
1 Identify poison, get victim to hospital urgently, and monitor victim regularly until help arrives. 2 Use a face mask or the mouth-to-nose method. 3 All of them. 4 Hypothermia may develop. 5 Lower the victim's body temperature by getting him to rest in a cool place. 6 Scrape it away with your fingernail or a rigid piece of plastic, such as a credit card. 7 Because they may squeeze more venom into the victim. 8 The swelling it causes can block the victim's airway. 9 Keep the victim still; keep her heart above the level of the bite; bandage above the bite. 10 Tetanus and rabies. 11 Get the victim to sit or lie down and cover the sting with an ice pack. 12 Pour lots of vinegar or ocean water over the wound, lightly cover the sting with a roller bandage, and call an ambulance.

Chapter 8 Medical problems and emergencies, page 139
1 A blockage in an artery carrying blood to part of the heart muscle. 2 That the victim will lose consciousness because the heart will stop beating (cardiac arrest). 3 a; c; e; and f. 4 Give the victim a sugary drink or something sweet to eat. 5 Breathing difficulties and loss of consciousness. 6 Autoinjector containing epinephrine. 7 a; b; c; and e. 8 Cool the victim by wiping the forehead with a cool, damp cloth and giving plenty of cool drinks. In addition, an adult may take two paracetamol tablets and a child the recommended dose of paracetamol syrup. 9 As illness starts: flu-like illness, high temperature, cold hands and feet, with limb pain, mottled skin. As infection develops: headache, stiff neck, vomiting, sensitivity to bright light, increasing drowsiness, distinctive rash. 10 Toothache; earache; abdominal pain.